THE JUICING DIET

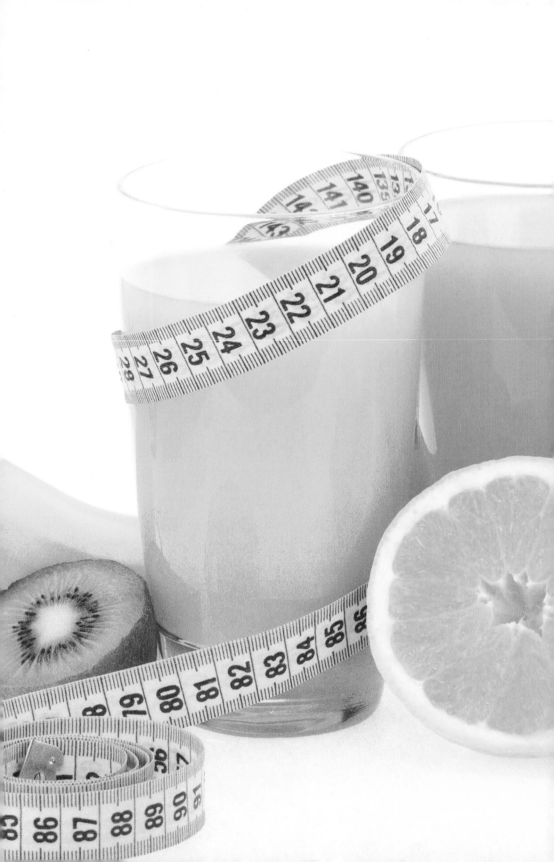

THE JUICING *DIET*

Drink Your Way to **WEIGHT LOSS, CLEANSING, HEALTH,** and **BEAUTY**

SONOMA PRESS

Contents

175 Healthful Juicing Recipes

Introduction

What would you say to someone who claimed to have consumed two cups of spinach, two carrots, a large stalk of celery, and a whole apple without taking a single bite?

What about someone who told you he or she took in an entire day's worth of vitamins and minerals in a single meal—a meal that wasn't significantly bigger than an average meal?

Would you believe it if someone told you he or she consumed more than 50 grams of healthful carbohydrates, protein, and fiber without taking in more than 2 or 3 grams of fat?

If none of these instances seem possible to you—or if they seem completely ridiculous—don't worry. You aren't going crazy; you simply may not be familiar with one of the latest trends in the world of health and fitness. Juicing has taken the wellness world by storm and is quickly gaining recognition as one of the simplest yet most beneficial changes you can make in your diet. All three of the claims made above can be realized in a single glass of fresh, home-pressed juice.

What is it about a fresh glass of juice in the morning that simultaneously quenches your thirst and wakes you up, making you ready to seize the day? While these effects may, to some degree, be psychological, there is a great deal of scientific evidence to support the idea that fresh juice is a healthful way to start the morning. Fresh juice is loaded with vitamins, minerals, and live enzymes that help nourish your body and keep it functioning at its optimal level. Not only is fresh juice a good source of nutrition, but it provides a number of other significant health benefits as well.

The juicing trend is sweeping the nation—it seems as though a new juice cleanse or detox hits the newsstands every few weeks. You may be tempted to think that juicing is just another fad diet, destined to fade along with the rest of them. The reality, however, is that the health claims associated with juicing have been supported by numerous medical studies. There are countless professionals in the medical and nutrition fields who support juicing as a means of supplementary nutrition.

With these facts in mind, you may find yourself making a trip to the grocery store to fill your cart with bottles of fruit and vegetable juice. Before you head to the checkout counter, consider this: bottled juices are pasteurized in a process that alters the juice nutritionally. In raw form, fruit and vegetable juices contain valuable vitamins, minerals, enzymes, and other nutrients that can be altered or destroyed through pasteurization. This affects the taste as well. If you've ever made your own fresh-squeezed orange juice at home, you've probably noticed how different it tastes from the stuff in a carton. Much of that difference can be attributed to those same vitamins, minerals, and enzymes that are destroyed in the pasteurization process. Why would you want to drink something that has had such a significant portion of its nutritional value chemically removed?

This is not to say that bottled juices are bad for you—they're simply a mediocre version of the real deal. Fresh-pressed juices are loaded with vitamins and minerals—not to mention authentic flavor—that can have a significant impact on your health and well-being. Numerous medical studies have provided evidence to support the idea that the consumption of raw juice helps boost the body's immune response, reduce the risk for chronic disease, and improve skin and hair health. Juicing has been associated with decreased inflammation, healthful weight loss, increased energy levels, and more. The results speak for themselves: juicing is a healthful way of life for anyone and everyone who is willing to give it a shot.

The Benefits of This Book

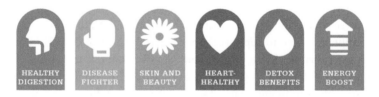

In this book you will learn the basics about what juicing is and how it can benefit you and your family, day to day and long-term. You'll also find 175 recipes for raw juice fit for any occasion; the juicing recipe icons (see the key above) will help you identify the top three health benefits of each of these delicious recipes. Whether you're looking for a simple snack or an on-the-go meal, these juices are sure to quench your thirst and give you an energy boost to power you through your day. The juicing wave is here—dive in!

The Basics of Juicing

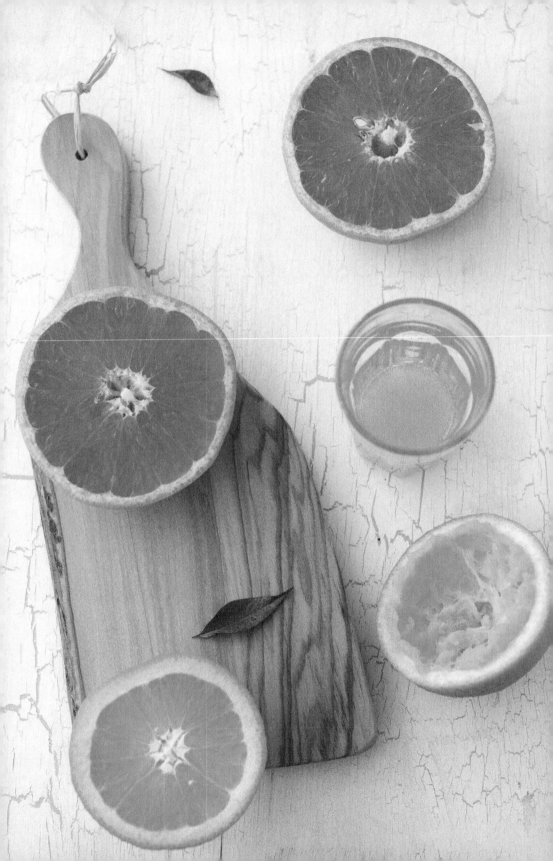

CHAPTER ONE

Getting Started with Juicing

Eating a diet with plenty of fruits and vegetables has been linked to improved health, and for good reason. Veggies and fruits…are loaded with vitamins, minerals, fiber, and antioxidants, which have been shown to protect against chronic diseases such as heart disease and cancer. They are also low in calories, making them a great choice for your waistline.

—DR. LISA R. YOUNG, *THE PORTION TELLER PLAN*

What Is Juicing?

The term "juicing" has a variety of different connotations. In this book, however, it's used to refer to the act of extracting liquid (juice) from plant tissues, including fresh fruits and vegetables. In the health and fitness world, "juicing" can also refer to the dietary habit of consuming nutrients and calories in the form of fresh-squeezed juice as an alternative or supplement to solid foods. This kind of juicing is often used in conjunction with detoxification and "cleanse" diets as a means of purging the body of accumulated toxins, replacing unwanted substances with healthful nutrients.

Juicing can be accomplished through a variety of means, both by hand and through the use of electronic appliances. Juicing by hand is also referred to as "hand squeezing" and is typically done using a juice press or citrus press (hand squeezing is most commonly used on citrus fruits). One of the most popular modern methods of juicing requires the use of a motor-driven device called, as you might expect, a juicer. These devices come in a variety of shapes and sizes, and they extract juice from plant foods through various methods, including mastication, shredding, grinding, and pressing.

In the next chapter you'll learn more about the various types of juicers to help you decide which type is right for you. But first, let's discuss the benefits of juicing, both practical and health-related.

Juicing Versus Eating Raw Vegetables

If you don't enjoy eating fresh fruits and vegetables, juicing may be a fun way to add them to your diet or to try fruits and vegetables you normally wouldn't eat.

—JENNIFER K. NELSON, RD, LD

If you aren't normally a fan of eating raw fruits and vegetables, don't assume that you won't enjoy juicing them. For some people, it's the texture that gets in the way. Some fruits have so much pulp or so many seeds that eating them can be a chore. Similarly, certain vegetables are difficult to eat without peeling, chopping, and cooking them. Juicing takes all the prep work out of the equation. It allows you to enjoy a refreshing beverage bursting with all of the flavor of fresh produce without any of the hassle.

In case you still aren't convinced that a glass full of liquid extracted from leafy green vegetables and celery stalks can be delicious, consider this: juicing lets you experiment with countless flavor combinations so you can find one that suits your preferences exactly. You don't have to stick to juicing just fruits or just vegetables, either—you can combine the two so the sweet flavor of your favorite fruit disguises the taste of vegetables you may not care for. Your eyes and brain may tell you that you're drinking a glass of liquefied broccoli and kale, but your taste buds will tell you that you are drinking a cool glass of apple juice.

Though juicing has a number of benefits over eating raw fruits and vegetables, there are a few things you need to keep in mind. The juicing process involves the extraction of juice from fresh produce by separating it from the skin, seeds, and pulp. These are the elements that contain the fiber, so by

NUTRITIONAL INFORMATION FOR FRESH KALE, BROCCOLI, AND APPLE JUICE

	KALE	BROCCOLI	APPLE	TOTAL
Serving Size	100 g	100 g	182 g	382 g
Calories	50	34	100	184
Protein	3 g	3 g	0 g	6 g
Carbs	10 g	7 g	25 g	42 g
Fat	1 g	0 g	0 g	1 g
Fiber	2 g	3 g	4 g	9 g
Vitamin C	200%	149%	14%	*
Calcium	14%	5%	2%	*
Iron	9%	4%	2%	*
Vitamin A	308%	12%	2%	*

* This value varies depending on your daily caloric intake.

removing them, you're also removing a significant portion of the fiber. A simple way to mitigate this loss, however, is to take a tablespoon or so of the pulp from your juicer's trap and stir it into your juice before drinking it.

The table above shows the nutritional content of a single glass of juice pressed from one serving each of fresh kale, broccoli, and apple.

Health Benefits of Juicing

Every person has the ability to reclaim all or some measure of their health. And every person who does that becomes a leader who inspires others.

—JOE CROSS, *FAT, SICK & NEARLY DEAD*

If you keep up with the latest health and fitness trends, you've probably already heard a little bit about juicing. You may have also heard that there is a great deal of debate over its health benefits. Some medical experts believe that juicing isn't significantly more nutritious than consuming whole fruits and vegetables. Others maintain that juicing provides unique health benefits that can't be obtained by consuming whole foods.

The biggest health benefit of juicing is you can greatly increase your daily intake of fresh fruits and vegetables without making major changes to your diet. Simply add a glass or two of fresh-squeezed juice into your daily routine. Of course, if you want to get the most benefit out of a juicing lifestyle, you should consider making some other healthful changes to your eating habits.

The following are some of the general health benefits of juicing:

- Nearly 95 percent of the enzymes and vitamins our bodies need can be found in raw juice. To obtain the same amount of nutrients as you would from a 16-ounce glass of juice, you would need to eat two pounds of carrots or a dozen apples.

- Juicing helps increase your daily energy levels, which may also help support weight-loss efforts.

- When consumed on an empty stomach, the nutrients in raw juice can be quickly absorbed by the body.

- Scientific evidence suggests that regular consumption of raw juice may help prevent chronic disease more effectively than vitamin supplements.

- Plant-based vitamins and minerals such as those found in raw juice are more easily absorbed and utilized by the body than synthetic vitamins and minerals.

- Raw juices contain beneficial live enzymes and natural antibiotics, which are often killed off during the pasteurization process for bottled juices.

The following are some of the benefits of choosing juicing over the consumption of whole fruits and vegetables:

- While there is little concrete evidence to suggest that raw juice is *healthier* than whole fruits and vegetables, it's easier to consume a glass of juice than a heaping portion of vegetables.

- It's easy to combine flavors of both fruits and vegetables in juice—you can disguise the flavors of foods you dislike with those you enjoy.

- Juice can be made from fruits and vegetables that are nearing their expiration date, when they may not be ideal for whole consumption.

- Often, you can juice the entire fruit or vegetable—no need to waste time peeling, coring, or chopping (you also get the nutrients found in the parts of the food you wouldn't normally eat).

- Proponents of juicing suggest that regular consumption of raw juice may help support a healthy digestive system. Even though some of the fiber content of the produce is lost, it takes less energy to digest liquid than solid food.

- If appearance or texture is an issue for you, juicing is a simple way to eliminate those obstacles. Even strange-looking foods like dragon fruit and mangosteen become delicious juice additives.

Though there may not be concrete evidence to suggest that drinking raw juice made from fresh produce is ultimately better for you than simply consuming whole fruits and vegetables, that doesn't make juicing any less healthful. As is true of all good dietary habits, it's all about how you make use of it. In moderation, drinking raw juices can be an excellent way to boost your daily nutrient intake if you tend not to eat a lot of raw fruits and vegetables. Instead, drink up!

Practical Benefits of Juicing

Juicing is more than just a method of improving your daily intake of healthful vitamins and minerals. It can also be a great option for a quick snack, a convenient way to feed your kids, and even a portable option for breakfast. The benefits of juicing go beyond health—it's extremely practical as well!

Some of the practical benefits associated with juicing include:

- A quick and easy process—it takes only a few minutes to prepare your fruits and vegetables, then juice them.

- Pulp extracted from fruits and vegetables can be used in recipes for baked goods or in soups and stews.

- Drinking homemade juice is a fast and simple way to boost your nutrient intake for the day without significantly increasing your daily calorie count.

- Homemade juice is a quick and easy option for a snack or an on-the-go meal for breakfast or lunch.

- You can use the leftover fruits and veggies your kids don't finish to create a healthful and nutritious snack for later.

- Juice is more filling than carbonated beverages and, depending on the ingredients you use, it can be much lower in calories.

- It's an easy way to work some vegetables into your diet, disguising the flavor with fresh fruits you enjoy.

- Juicing enables you to use the whole fruit or vegetable—save the stalks from large heads of broccoli for use in your next glass of juice, instead of throwing them out.

- Homemade juice will help keep you hydrated during the day if you tend not to drink a lot of water.

- Juicing is an easy way to use the produce in your fridge that is getting ready to spoil—don't waste money!

- It's a great way to take advantage of seasonal produce and low-cost fruits and vegetables at local farmers' markets.

Once you start juicing on your own, you'll discover a number of other benefits that will have you wondering why you didn't start juicing sooner!

How to Make Your Own Juice

Making your own homemade juice is incredibly easy. You should still wash your fruits and vegetables as you normally would, but generally, you don't need to peel or chop them. Certain foods may be too large to fit into the juicer's chute whole, in which case you may need to trim the food or cut it in half or in quarters so it will fit. After preparing your produce, simply place a pitcher or container under the juicer's spout; then feed the produce through the chute.

Making Homemade Juice

1. Purchase fresh produce.

2. Rinse and trim produce as needed to fit in juicer.

3. Feed produce through the juicer.

4. Enjoy delicious, freshly pressed juice.

5. Repeat!

Tips for Juicing at Home

With the right mind-set and the proper equipment, juicing at home can be incredibly easy. There are, however, right and wrong ways to go about it. Before you begin juicing, take the time to read through these tips to make sure you get the most out of your new juicer.

- Rinse your fruit and vegetable ingredients well before juicing—this will help remove dirt or pesticides that may be on the food.

- Remember that raw juice is perishable—the longer you wait to drink it, the less nutritional benefit you'll receive (it's best to drink raw juice right away, but you can store it in the fridge for up to three days).

- If you must store raw juice, put it in an airtight glass container and fill the container to the top to avoid oxidization.

- When using citrus fruits in raw juices, remove the peel but retain as much as you can of the white pith just below the skin.

- To make juicing leafy greens easier, roll them into a ball before feeding them through your juicer.

- Add a fresh apple or pear to your vegetable juice to sweeten it up and disguise the flavor of bitter greens.

- Keep in mind that certain fruit and vegetable ingredients provide certain benefits. Consult the appendices for details about individual ingredients.

- Don't be afraid to add fresh herbs and spices to your juices. A little bit of fresh cilantro can brighten up your juice, while an inch of fresh ginger can provide a deep, more savory flavor.

- To increase your daily intake of heart-healthful fats, drizzle a teaspoon of coconut oil into your juice.

- Avoid drinking large quantities of citrus-based juices in the morning to reduce stomach cramps—the acid in these juices can cause reflux.

- Cucumbers are a great base for raw juice because they have a high water content and a mild flavor.

- Always rinse your juicer immediately after using it—the longer you wait to clean it, the more difficult the task will be.

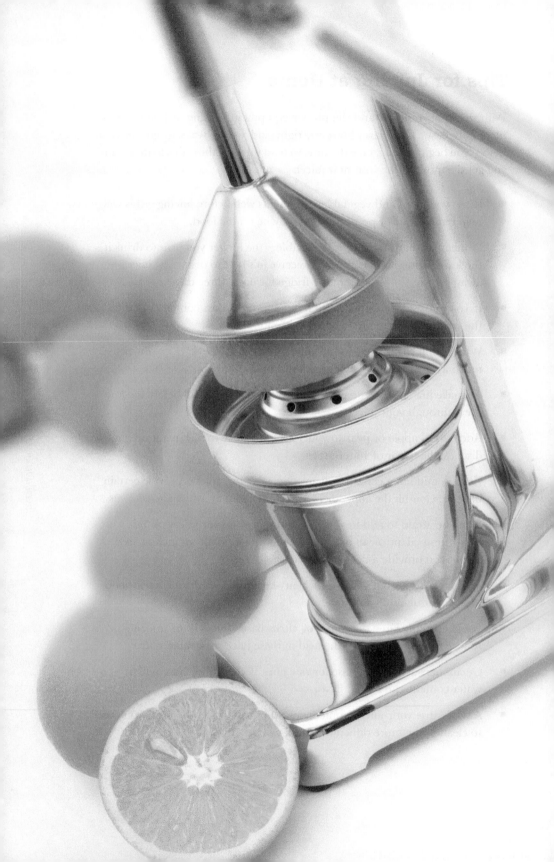

CHAPTER TWO

Juicer Buyer's Guide

The juices extracted from fresh raw vegetables and fruits are the means by which we can furnish all the cells and tissues of the body with the elements and nutritional enzymes they need in the manner they can be most readily digested and assimilated.

—DR. NORMAN WALKER

When it comes to buying a juicer, you may be overwhelmed at first by the sheer number of options. Masticating juicers, twin-gear juicers, centrifugal juice extractors—how can you even tell them apart? Not all juicers are created equal, but there isn't necessarily one type or model that's "best"; it all depends on your own needs and preferences. In this chapter you'll learn about the different types of juicers and get some valuable tips for finding and purchasing a juicer for yourself or your family.

Different Types of Juicers

Juicers are often broken down into three main categories: centrifugal, masticating, and triturating. Within these categories, however, there are a few variations. Below you'll find explanations of six different kinds of juicers, including details about what foods they are recommended for as well as their advantages and disadvantages over other types of juicers.

Non-Ejection Centrifugal Juicer

Perhaps one of the most basic types of juicer, non-ejection centrifugal juicers are typically recommended for producing juice to feed one or two people, not a large family. This type of juicer works by spinning a shredder disc at high speed. As fruits and vegetables are fed into the machine, the ingredients come into contact with the disc and are shredded into pulp. The juice passes through holes in the stainless steel shredder basket and exits the machine through a spout in the front. The disadvantage of this type of juicer is that it can produce only about one quart of juice at a time before it must be stopped and the shredder basket cleaned.

Automatic-Ejection Centrifugal Juicer

An automatic-ejection centrifugal juicer operates in a way very similar to the centrifugal juicer already mentioned. The main difference, and key advantage of this type of juicer, is that you don't need to stop and clean the machine before you're finished juicing. As ingredients are inserted into the juicer, they still come into contact with the shredder basket and are ground into pulp. The pulp, however, is then deposited into a canister in the back of the juicer. Automatic-ejection centrifugal juicers are also available with extra-large feeding chutes to accommodate larger ingredients. With a three-inch-diameter feeding chute, you don't have to waste time chopping ingredients before you start juicing.

Single-Gear Juicer (Masticating Juicer)

Also called a masticating juicer, a single-gear juicer is newer than the centrifugal juicer and provides some unique benefits. It operates at a much slower speed, which helps reduce friction and heat, thus preserving more of the original nutrient content of the ingredients. Masticating juicers work by rotating an auger at a rate of around 80 rpm, squeezing and pressing the fruit and vegetables forward through the juicer. As the ingredients are pressed, the juice flows into one receptacle while the pulp flows into a separate one. Another benefit of this type of juicer is that it's fairly easy to clean.

Upright Masticating Juicer

Upright masticating juicers are a relatively new design. They combine the low-speed and low-heat benefits of traditional single-gear juicers with a more contemporary, space-saving upright design. These models actually press the juice twice, which increases the yield. As the juice is extracted, the resulting pulp is pressed again before being ejected. This results in a drier pulp and a higher yield of fresh juice. Masticating juicers are also very versatile as compared with other models—they can be used to make baby food, nut butters, desserts from frozen fruit, and pasta shapes out of fresh vegetables like zucchini.

Twin-Gear Juicer (Triturating Juicer)

The most expensive type of juicer is the twin-gear or triturating juicer. These juicers operate at an even slower speed than masticating juicers, resulting in even less oxidation and nutrient destruction. Juices made using a twin-gear juicer also have a longer shelf life because the low operating speed means that there is less oxygen in the resulting juice. These juicers work by forcing fruit and vegetable ingredients through two interlocking roller gears. The pressure created by the gears breaks open the cell walls, releasing not only the juice itself but also the enzymes, vitamins, and trace minerals. These juicers are capable of juicing nearly any kind of plant material, including pine needles, wheatgrass, and more.

Wheatgrass Juicer

A wheatgrass juicer is exactly what it sounds like: a type of juicer made exclusively for juicing wheatgrass. This type of juicer can also be used to juice other leafy greens and some soft fruits such as grapes, but they cannot handle hard or dense fruits and vegetables like other juicers can. Wheatgrass juicers come in both manual and electric models.

Cold-Pressed Versus Centrifugal

Centrifugal juicers are some of the most popular models on the market because they're affordable and easy to use. These juicers can handle most types of fruits and vegetables commonly used for juicing, and they create juice fairly quickly. Their major disadvantage is that they utilize a shredder basket or strainer screen to separate the pulp from the juice; this basket or screen spins very quickly inside the juicer, which creates the centrifugal force needed to extract the juice from the pulp. The speed of the basket also creates heat and friction, however, which destroys part of the nutrient content of the juice before it even exits the juicer.

Due to the heat involved in the juicing process using centrifugal juicers, the shelf life of the juice is fairly low. As the juice is extracted from the ingredients, it's aerated and the oxygen bubbles dissolved in the juice cause it to spoil fairly quickly. Juice made using a centrifugal juicer is best consumed immediately, because even if you store it for only a few hours, it could lose a significant portion of its nutritional value in that time. Another disadvantage of centrifugal juicers is that the pulp extracted from the fresh ingredients is still wet, meaning that there is more juice that could be extracted but, unfortunately, goes to waste.

Masticating juicers are often referred to as cold-press juicers because they don't produce the same heat for which centrifugal juicers are known. One of the highest-quality cold-press juicers on the market is the Norwalk Juicer. This juicer works by creating a tremendous amount of pressure using a hydraulic press. The juice is extracted through this intense pressure, rather than through shredding or grinding, so its natural vitamins, minerals, and trace elements are preserved. The flavor of cold-pressed juice is also generally considered to be greatly superior to that of centrifugal juicers. Cold-pressed juicers also have the benefit of creating a higher yield because the juice is literally forced out of the pulp, leaving very little behind.

Where to Buy a Juicer

The type of juicer you buy is more important than where you buy it, but if you want to get the most bang for your buck, you should do a little price comparison. Because juicing has become so popular lately, buying a juicer is easier than ever. You can find juicers in the home section of most major department stores as well as some electronics and appliance stores, including Best Buy and H.H. Gregg. You can also find them at home and kitchen stores such as Bed Bath & Beyond.

Another great option to find a juicer is to look online. Websites like Amazon and eBay are great places to find new and gently used appliances for the home and kitchen. One benefit of Amazon over eBay is that you're likely to find a larger selection of new products offered from manufacturers or wholesalers rather than individual sellers. Take the time to shop around both online and in store to find the best price you can.

Choosing the Right Juicer for You

When it comes to choosing a juicer, it's all about comparing the pros and cons. Consider the amount of time you have to spend juicing each day and how important it is to you that the device be easy to clean. You should also consider whether oxidation and heat production are significant problems for you or if you simply want to be able to quickly make a glass of fresh juice in the morning. This list should help you narrow down your options.

Centrifugal Juicer

Pros:

- Ideal for one or two people

- Can handle a variety of fruits and vegetables

- One of the fastest models

- Most affordable type of juicer

Cons:

- Centrifugal force, which creates heat/friction that results in loss of some nutritional content

- Oxidation, which decreases shelf life

- Not ideal for leafy greens

- More waste than other models

Cold-Press Juicer (Masticating Juicer)

Pros:

- Slower juicing process, higher quality of juice

- Less heat/friction, meaning fewer nutrients lost

- Ideal for most vegetables, including leafy greens

- Juice with longer shelf life

- Less waste

Cons:

- Slower to operate than many models
- Can be very expensive
- May take up more shelf/counter space

Citrus Juicer

Pros:

- Simplest type of juicer, easy to use
- Ideal for juicing oranges, lemons, and other citrus fruits
- May be manual or electric

Cons:

- Considerably varied construction quality
- Can juice only citrus fruits
- May not have variable pulp control

Twin-Gear Juicer (Triturating Juicer)

Pros:

- Slow rpm, preserving more nutrients
- Twin-gear process, which extracts maximum amount of juice
- Higher quality juice
- Ideal for leafy greens, root vegetables, and wheatgrass

Cons:

- More expensive than many models
- Slower to operate
- Takes more time to clean

Wheatgrass Juicer

Pros:

- Ideal for juicing wheatgrass

- Can also juice leafy greens and soft fruits like grapes

- Comes in manual or electric form

Cons:

- Not ideal for juicing most fruits and vegetables

Know which juicer's best for you? Great! In the next section, you'll learn what to put in it.

PART TWO

The Ingredients

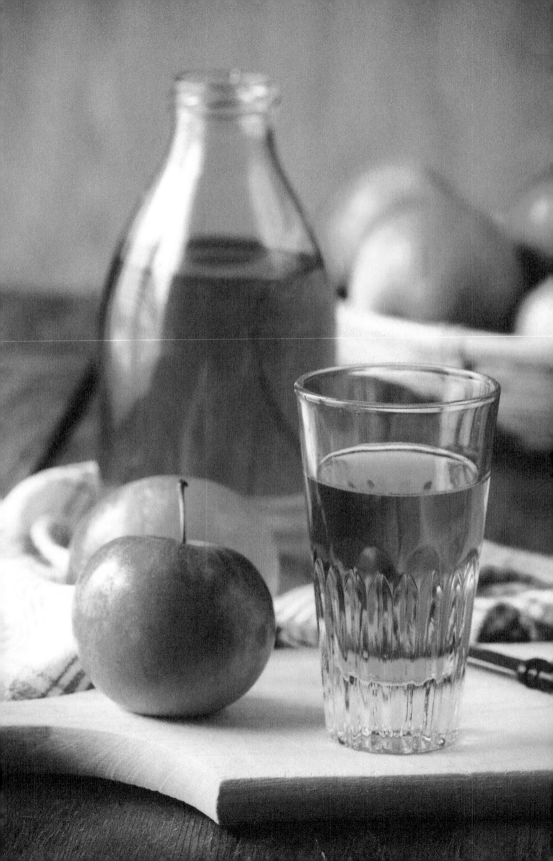

CHAPTER THREE

35 Fruits Perfect for Juicing

Nature has provided us with the finest fruits and vegetables, each designed to prevent and heal disease, whilst at the same time feeding every single cell in the body. Although every fruit and vegetable comes in a solid protective layer, it is the juice contained within [their] fibers...which ultimately feeds the body.

—JASON VALE, JUICE MASTER USA

To get the most out of your juices, you need to think carefully about the ingredients you put into them. Fresh fruits and vegetables offer a variety of health benefits that can help relieve common ailments, improve chronic conditions, and increase your overall health. In this chapter you'll receive basic info about juicing fruit at home.

35 Fruits to Try

These healthful, great-tasting fruits are perfect in juice:

- Apple
- Apricot
- Blackberries
- Blood orange
- Blueberries
- Cantaloupe
- Cherries
- Cranberries
- Figs
- Gooseberries
- Grapes
- Grapefruit
- Guava
- Honeydew
- Jicama
- Kiwi
- Kumquat
- Lemon

- Lime
- Mango
- Nectarine
- Orange
- Papaya
- Passion fruit
- Peach
- Pear
- Persimmon
- Pineapple
- Plum
- Pomegranate
- Raspberries
- Starfruit
- Strawberries
- Tangerine
- Watermelon

Benefits of Juicing Fruit

For many people, gulping down a glass of cold orange juice is the best way to wake up in the morning. But what is it about that cold glass of juice that tastes so refreshing and revitalizing? Perhaps it is the acidity of the citrus or the fresh fruit flavor. It could also be the numerous vitamins and minerals that get your blood flowing and your brain working. Regardless of your personal reasons for drinking juice, fruit juices provide a number of significant benefits, including:

- Unique flavors that can disguise the bitterness of vegetable ingredients

- Healthful blends of vitamins and minerals

- Live enzymes that provide numerous benefits for the body

- Sweetness to help contrast other strong flavors

- A wide variety of flavors to choose from

- High levels of antioxidants

- Unique flavors when used alone or in combination

- A full serving of fruit in each 4-ounce glass of fruit juice

- A great source of vitamin C, potassium, and folate

- Helping improve the health of skin, hair, and nails

- Boosting immune response and preventing disease

Cautions and Caveats

Though fresh fruits add delicious flavor and texture to raw juices, there are a few things to bear in mind. The most significant caveat of using fruits in raw juice is that fruit juice has a higher calorie content than most vegetables. For many people, juicing is about losing weight and improving overall health. If your goal is to reduce your daily calorie intake in order to lose weight, you may need to limit the amount of fruit juice you drink. Because juice is naturally less filling than solid food, it's easy to take in a significant number of calories in a short period of time.

It's also important to realize that while juicing fresh fruits is a wonderful way to increase your daily intake of vital nutrients, it shouldn't completely replace the consumption of whole fruits. The juicing process does exactly what it implies—it extracts the juice from the fruit. This means that you get all of the delicious flavor of those tart apples and ripe berries, but you miss out on the healthful nutrients contained in the skin of the fruit. Not only is the skin a valuable source of dietary fiber, it can also contain key nutrients that you may not be able to get from juice alone. This is not to say that drinking fruit juice is bad for you—you simply need to remember that drinking fruit juice should be a supplement to consuming whole fruits, not a replacement.

Simple Ways to Incorporate Fruit

There are many ways to incorporate fruit into your raw juices—it all depends whether you want the fruit to complement the other ingredient or be the star of the recipe. In recipes where you just want a little bit of sweetness, add a ripe pear or apple. For times when you need a strong flavor to disguise the bitterness of dandelion greens or Brussels sprouts, try adding a handful of strawberries or a citrus fruit with strong flavor. If you want to encourage your children to drink raw juices, fruit will be instrumental in disguising both the color and flavor of vegetables. Picky eaters may refuse to drink anything that looks even remotely like a vegetable, so brightly colored fruits like raspberries and blueberries may help cover up that telltale green vegetable color.

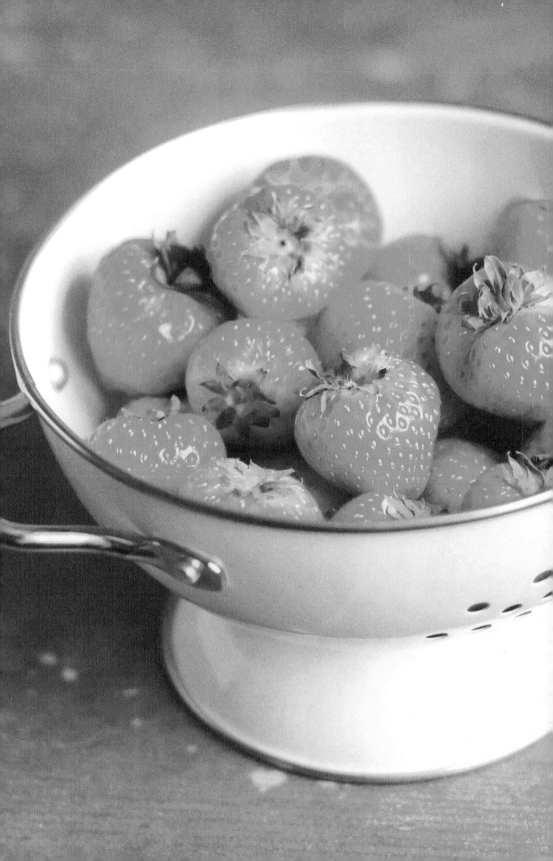

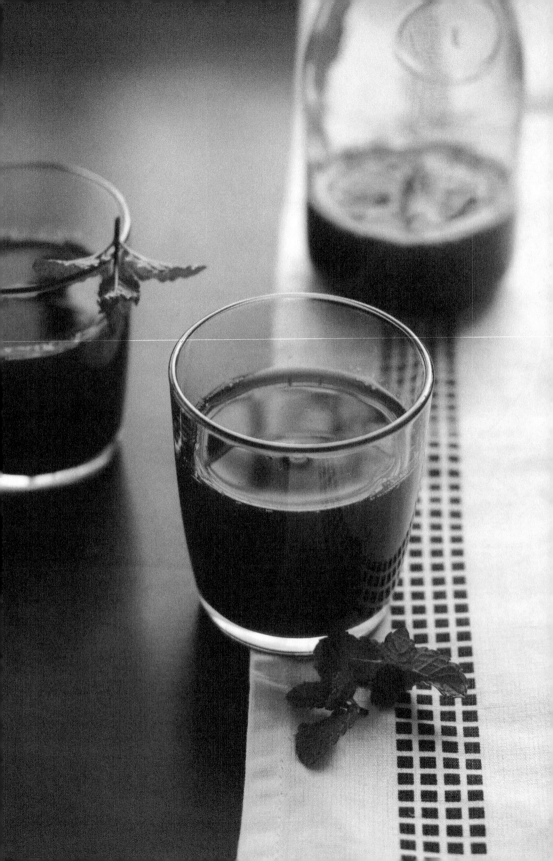

CHAPTER FOUR

35 Vegetables Perfect for Juicing

If you're not big into fruits and vegetables, it's a good way to get them in. It can help you meet daily recommendations in one drink.

—JENNIFER BARR, MPH, RD, LDN

If your children are like most, getting them to eat their vegetables can be quite a challenge. You might even have a tendency to avoid anything green or leafy yourself. But it's important to realize that vegetables are a vital source of healthful minerals, vitamins, and enzymes that your body needs to run properly. In this section you'll learn the basics about thirty-five different vegetables that can easily be incorporated into homemade juices to increase your daily nutrient intake.

35 Vegetables to Try

Experiment with these vegetable powerhouses:

- Arugula
- Asparagus
- Beets
- Bell pepper
- Bok choy
- Broccoli
- Brussels sprouts
- Cabbage
- Carrots
- Cauliflower
- Celeriac
- Celery
- Collard greens
- Cucumber
- Dandelion greens
- Kale
- Kohlrabi
- Mustard greens
- Onion
- Parsnips
- Pumpkin
- Radishes
- Romaine lettuce
- Rutabaga
- Scallions
- Spinach
- Sugar snap peas
- Summer squash
- Sweet potato
- Swiss chard
- Tomatoes
- Turnips
- Turnip greens
- Wheatgrass
- Zucchini

Benefits of Vegetables for Juicing

Fresh vegetables are packed with vitamins, minerals, and other nutrients. However, some nutrients are better absorbed by your body after they've been cooked. This is true of tomatoes, for example, and some nutrients, including vitamins A, E, and K, are not easily digestible in juice form. To get the most benefit out of your vegetable juices, you need to learn which vegetables have readily digestible nutrients so you can power-pack your recipes. Some of the best vegetables to use for nutrient-rich juices include leafy greens, red peppers, broccoli, and asparagus. Try to incorporate at least a handful of one of these ingredients in every recipe to fill out the nutrient profile.

The beauty of vegetables for juicing is that they are so incredibly varied—not only does each vegetable have its own unique flavor, but they also contain a variety of nutrients. Beets, for example, can help lower blood pressure, while cucumbers are packed with potassium, and carrots help reduce the risk of cardiovascular disease. In the appendices at the end of this book you'll find an in-depth nutrient profile for each of the fruit and vegetable ingredients covered in this section. By familiarizing yourself with the health benefits of individual ingredients, you can create custom recipes to provide your body with the nutrients it needs most.

Cautions and Caveats

Fortunately, most vegetables have a lower calorie count per serving than most fruits do. This being the case, calorie content is not as much of a concern with vegetable-based juices as it is with fruits. Your major cause for concern with vegetable juices may be the flavor. If you're not a fan of raw vegetables, you may find vegetable-based juices hard to stomach at first. The key is to start with some of the more subtle vegetable flavors until you get used to it. Then you can begin to experiment with bolder flavors, mellowing them out with some fruit if you need to.

Another great way to counteract the strong flavor of some vegetables is to experiment with a few additives. Fresh herbs, spices, and other supplements can transform both the flavor and the nutrient content of raw vegetable juices. Even a dash of cinnamon or cayenne pepper can change the whole flavor profile of your juice. In the next chapter you'll learn about a large assortment of additives that can help you achieve flavors you'll come to crave in your homemade raw juices.

Simple Ways to Incorporate Vegetables

As you've already discovered, vegetables are an excellent source of dietary fiber and a wide variety of vitamins and minerals. Just a handful of spinach or kale can greatly increase the nutrient content of your juice, so why not throw some in? Even if you prefer fruit-based juices, you can still incorporate vegetables in a very simple and nearly undetectable way. For example, blending a few sprigs of fresh mint or cilantro into a glass of fruit juice will up the nutrient content while also helping boost the fresh, clean flavor of your juice. Even a handful of a strong-flavored vegetable like collard greens or broccoli may go unnoticed in a fruit-based juice.

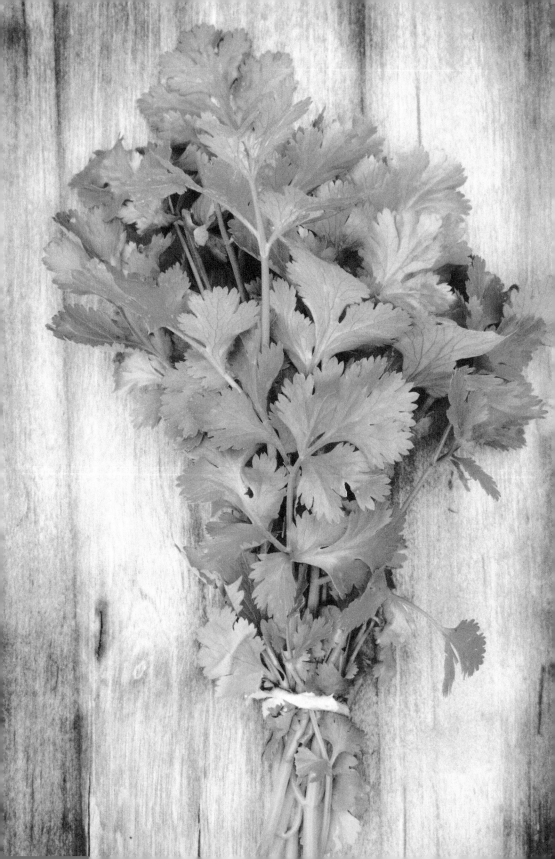

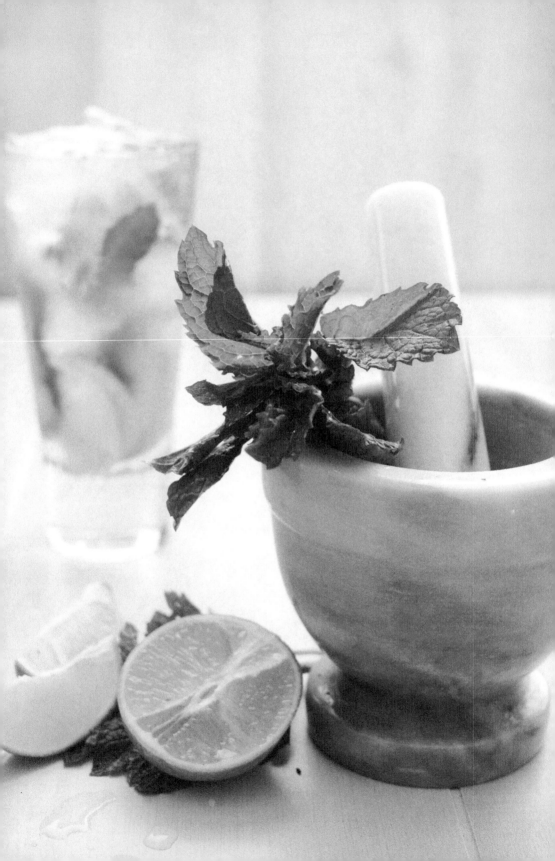

CHAPTER FIVE

Supplements, Herbs, and Spices for Juicing

Using herbs can be very beneficial for your health. Herbs come in many forms...fresh, dried, in tinctures, and dried powders. The good news is, you can use them in any of these forms by adding them to your juice!

—VANESSA SIMKINS, *THE JUICING MIXOLOGIST*

In addition to the fruits and vegetables already listed, you can also incorporate a variety of supplements, herbs, and spices into your homemade juices. These ingredients can greatly increase the nutritional value of your juices while also enhancing the flavor. A dash of ground cinnamon or a handful of fresh basil leaves can significantly change the flavor of your homemade juice. In this chapter you'll learn about the health benefits associated with some of the most popular supplements, herbs, and spices for juicing as well as recommendations for how to use them.

Popular Supplements for Juicing

There are a wide variety of supplements that can be incorporated into juicing for several different purposes. Supplements may take the form of powders, tinctures, oils, seeds, and more. Each supplement serves a unique purpose, and you can use them to customize your juicing recipes to suit your needs. Some of the most popular supplements for juicing include:

- Aloe vera
- Apple cider vinegar
- Bee pollen
- Chia seeds
- Chlorella
- Coconut oil
- Flaxseed
- Hemp seed
- Kudzu

- Nutritional yeast
- Nuts
- Omega-3
- Probiotics
- Sea buckthorn
- Spirulina
- Stevia
- Vitamin B_{12}
- Wheatgrass powder

Aloe Vera

Aloe vera is a green succulent plant belonging to the lily family. Though commonly associated with sunburn relief, aloe vera actually has a number of benefits to offer. The juice of the aloe vera plant contains more than two hundred different vitamins and minerals as well as essential fatty acids, enzymes, and amino acids. Adding aloe vera juice to your raw juices may help improve your body's ability to fight disease, aid your digestion, and help improve your cardiovascular health.

Apple Cider Vinegar

Apple cider vinegar probably makes you think about pickles or salad dressing, not juice. Raw, unfiltered apple cider vinegar is, however, an excellent ingredient for raw juice because it's loaded with health benefits. Not only does apple cider vinegar have an antiseptic effect that can reduce breath odor but it also helps your skin look more firm and youthful. Apple cider vinegar also helps soothe stomach irritation, prevent indigestion, get rid of congestion, and relieve sore throats.

Bee Pollen

Bee pollen may seem like a strange ingredient to add to juice, but a research study conducted by the San Francisco Medical Research Foundation suggests that bee pollen contains more than five thousand different enzymes and co-enzymes—more than any other food. Some of the nutrients found in bee pollen include digestion-aiding enzymes like catalase and amylase as well as vitamin B_{12}, essential amino acids, essential fatty acids, and complex carbohydrates. Many of the vitamins and other nutrients found in bee pollen are already predigested, which makes them easy for the body to absorb.

Chia Seeds

Chia seeds may not look like anything but tiny brown specks, but they're actually packed with nutrients. These seeds are derived from a flowering plant that belongs to the mint family and are associated with a number of health benefits, including lowered cholesterol, stabilized blood sugar levels, improved digestion, and higher energy levels. Some of the other benefits linked to chia seeds include reduced risk for diabetes, increased fiber intake, stronger teeth and bones, improved insulin response, and appetite regulation.

Chlorella

Chlorella is a type of algae that is known for its high protein content. This algae contains 5 grams of protein per teaspoon, so adding a full tablespoon or two to a glass of fresh juice can go a long way toward meeting your daily protein requirements. Chlorella is particularly recommended as a supplement for pregnant women because it contains chlorella growth factor, a type of anabolic energy that has been shown to support the growth of the fetus. This supplement can be combined with spirulina in fresh juice.

Coconut Oil

If you've never used coconut oil before, you're missing out on a wealth of valuable benefits. By weight, coconut oil has the lowest calorie count of nearly all fat sources. In addition, it contains medium-chain rather than long-chain fatty acids, which are digested more readily as a source of energy. Coconut oil also helps you burn fat, stave off infections, reduce hunger, and regulate blood cholesterol levels. Stir a teaspoon of coconut oil into your fresh juice to feel the benefits!

Flaxseed

Flaxseed has often been referred to as a "super food" because it contains some serious health benefits. It's been linked to reduced risk for chronic diseases like diabetes and some forms of cancer, and has also been shown to lower blood pressure, which helps prevent heart disease. Some of the other benefits associated with flaxseed include reduced inflammation, lower cholesterol levels, and relief from hot flashes. Flaxseed is also a good source of fiber, not to mention omega-3 fatty acids.

Hemp Seed

When you hear the word "hemp," you may picture flowing prairie skirts or tie-dyed tunics. Hemp seed is actually a powerful, health-boosting ingredient that works very well in fresh juice and is rich in protein. Not only does hemp seed contain protein, but the type of protein it contains is easy to digest—unlike some seeds and other protein sources, it doesn't cause bloating or gas.

Kudzu

Kudzu is a type of Chinese herb, also called *Pueraria lobata*. It is technically a vine, the root, flower, and leaves of which are used to make a medicinal powder. In ancient China, kudzu was used to treat alcoholism, but today it's used to relieve headaches, dizziness, and upset stomach. It has also been used to treat the symptoms of menopause, fever, diarrhea, and measles.

Nutritional Yeast

Unless you're a vegan or vegetarian, you may not be familiar with nutritional yeast. This substance is a type of deactivated yeast, typically sold in flakes or powder as a condiment or an ingredient in recipes. Nutritional yeast is an excellent source of vegan and vegetarian protein. It also contains a number of essential vitamins and minerals, including vitamin B_{12}, selenium, potassium, and iron.

Nuts

Nuts may seem like a strange ingredient to add to fresh juice, but they can taste great and improve your health. One of the best ways to use nuts in your fresh juice is to grind the raw nuts into a powder, and then sprinkle it on top or stir it into your juice. Many nuts, like walnuts and almonds, contain unsaturated fatty acids that may help reduce your blood cholesterol levels and your risk for heart disease. Nuts also contain omega-3 fatty acids, fiber, and a variety of minerals and vitamins like vitamin E.

Omega-3

Omega-3, or fish oil supplements, make a great addition to homemade juice. Omega-3 is good for just about everyone, especially those with heart disease. Its benefits include reduced blood pressure, regulated blood sugar levels, reduced risk for heart attack and stroke, and even slowed development of plaque in the arteries. The human body doesn't produce omega-3 fatty acid, so it's a good idea to take a supplement once in a while, especially if you don't eat a lot of fish.

Probiotics

If you've ever seen a commercial for yogurt, you're probably familiar with the term "probiotic." Probiotics are live bacteria that help regulate and improve digestion. Unlike some bacteria that may cause infections and make you sick, probiotics are good bacteria that your body needs to function properly. To increase your intake of probiotics, open a probiotic capsule and stir half or all of the contents into a glass of fresh juice and enjoy.

Sea Buckthorn

Sea buckthorn (*Hippophae rhamnoides*) typically comes in capsules that can be opened and stirred into your juice. It contains palmitoleic acid, a type of fatty acid that's found naturally in human skin. This acid helps moisturize and heal the skin. It is particularly effective for hydrating mucous membranes and for alleviating vaginal dryness.

Spirulina

Spirulina is a type of blue-green algae known for its high concentration of nontoxic, absorbable nutrients. This supplement is a surprising substitute for protein powder because it contains all eight essential amino acids, making it a complete protein. Spirulina is also a good source of vital nutrients, including vitamins A, E, and K as well as trace minerals, phytonutrients, and enzymes. Spirulina is typically available in flake or powder form. Simply add one or two tablespoons to your fresh juice.

Stevia

Stevia is a calorie-free sweetener derived from a plant belonging to the sunflower family. This sweetener is preferred by many over traditional sugar because it's "natural," not to mention the fact that it has no calories. Studies of the stevia plant have revealed compounds that have anti-inflammatory, anti-tumor, diuretic, and anti-hypertensive properties. For many people, however, stirring a little stevia into a glass of homemade juice is just an easy and guilt-free way to sweeten it up.

Vitamin B$_{12}$

Vitamin B$_{12}$ can't be produced by the human body—which is why B$_{12}$ supplements are so popular. It can be found in meat, fish, and dairy. It can also be made in a laboratory, as an option for individuals following a vegan or vegetarian diet. Some of its benefits include improved memory and concentration, slowed aging, reduced risk for diabetes, relief from depression and sleep disorders, reduced inflammation, and improved immune system health.

Wheatgrass Powder

Wheatgrass is derived from the same wheat used to produce flour—it's simply harvested while the plant is still small and green. The leaves of the plant can be juiced fresh or added to fresh juice in powdered form. One of the benefits of wheatgrass is that, despite being derived from wheat, it doesn't contain any gluten, making it safe for those suffering from celiac disease or gluten intolerance. Wheatgrass contains a variety of amino acids, vitamins, and enzymes, including chlorophyll, which helps oxygenate the blood and detoxify the body.

Healthful Herbs for Juicing

You may be surprised to learn that several simple herbs actually contain amazing healing powers. Numerous studies have linked the consumption of fresh herbs to reduced risk for chronic disease, relief from migraines, reversal of heart disease, and improved insulin response in diabetics. Fresh herbs can also help to detoxify, strengthen, and purify the body. In addition to these health benefits, they're delicious. Cilantro, for example, can give any juice a boost of freshness, while sweet basil and oregano lend a more savory flavor. Some of the most popular herbs for juicing include:

- Andrographis
- Basil
- Cilantro
- Coriander
- Dill
- Echinacea
- Lavender
- Mint

- Oregano
- Parsley
- Peppermint
- Rosemary
- Sage
- St. John's wort
- Thyme

Andrographis

This herb is not as well known as some others, but it still contains some significant beneficial properties. Andrographis has been shown to help ease the symptoms of fatigue and sleeplessness. It may also help relieve sore throats and runny nose. These properties make Andrographis a must-have additive if you're suffering from a cold or sinusitis.

Basil

Basil is a leafy green herb often used to flavor pasta sauce and other Italian-style dishes. You may be surprised to hear, however, that it can also fight stress and disease. Studies on mice revealed that a tea made from basil leaves may help shrink tumors by reducing their blood supply and thus stopping their spread. Basil has also been shown to have anti-inflammatory and antibacterial properties. It may also help reduce the risk for cardiovascular disease by protecting cells from free radical damage.

Cilantro

Cilantro has a wonderful fresh flavor that works well in either vegetable or fruit juices. It's rich in antioxidants and has also been found to work as a digestive aid and an antibacterial agent. Cilantro is a good source of dietary fiber, essential oils, and a variety of vitamins. It's been shown to reduce cholesterol levels, to aid in red blood cell production, and to help prevent bone loss.

Coriander

Coriander is the name for the seed derived from the cilantro plant. These seeds can be used in either fresh or dried form, and they provide a number of significant health benefits. Coriander seed is best known for its anti-diabetic properties—it helps control blood sugar and cholesterol levels while also limiting the production of damaging free radicals. Coriander is also a very phytonutrient-rich herb, containing a variety of flavonoids and active phenolic acid compounds.

Dill

Dill has a tangy taste that is often used in summer recipes for salads and soups. This herb contains two different types of healing compounds: monoterpenes and flavonoids. Monoterpenes, like carvone, anethofuran, and limonene, provide antibacterial benefits; according to recent studies, they may also provide anti-cancer benefits. Flavonoids like vicenin and kaempferol may help reduce inflammation, protect blood vessels, and prevent free radical damage. Dill has also been shown to help prevent bone loss by helping the body absorb calcium more easily.

Echinacea

Echinacea purpurea, or the purple coneflower, is commonly used as an herbal remedy against colds and the flu. This herb helps protect white blood cells and has been shown to boost the immune system, aiding the body as it fights off illness. Though it's been proven to reduce the risk for colds by as much as 50 percent in some individuals, it can have some side effects. Echinacea may trigger asthma in very sensitive individuals and may also interact with some medications.

Lavender

Lavender can be used in a variety of ways. The fresh flowers and leaves can be incorporated into juice, the herb can be dried, or you can use lavender essential oil. No matter which way you choose to use this herb, it's rich in medicinal benefits. Lavender has a calming effect, which is excellent for anxiety issues. It can also be used to treat migraines, depression, and emotional stress. This herb is also known as an alternative treatment for insomnia, because it has been shown to improve sleep patterns. In addition to these benefits, lavender has also been used as an acne treatment, a bug repellent, a diuretic, and a pain reliever.

Mint

Mint has been associated with a number of medical benefits, including relief from cramping, bloating, diarrhea, and the symptoms of irritable bowel syndrome. It contains menthol, which helps relax the muscles by blocking the flow of calcium, which causes them to contract. Mint has also been shown to improve skin health and digestion, and to relieve minor aches and pains, headaches, and congestion.

Oregano

Oregano is very popular in cooking for its aromatic flavor. It's a great source of vitamin K and it also contains a variety of antioxidants. Fresh oregano is incredibly nutrient-dense and an excellent source of fiber. Perhaps one of the most significant benefits of this herb, however, is the fact that it contains volatile oils like thymol and carvacrol. Both of these oils have been shown to inhibit bacterial growth. In fact, oregano has been found to be more effective against Giardia than most medications prescribed for the disease.

Parsley

Often used as an ingredient in soups or a garnish for dishes in a variety of cuisines, parsley makes an excellent addition to fresh juice. This herb contains more than 150 percent of your daily recommended intake for vitamin K and more than 16 percent of your daily dose of vitamin C. Parsley contains a number of volatile oils that have been shown to reduce tumor formation and to neutralize certain types of carcinogens. It's also rich in antioxidants, which help oxygenate the blood and prevent and repair damage caused by free radicals.

Peppermint

In addition to its iconic flavor, peppermint is also known as a remedy for gas and upset stomach. Peppermint is believed to provide these benefits because it relaxes the muscles in the gut. It's loaded with nutrients that help improve digestion and skin complexion, prevent cancer, and relieve the symptoms of colds and the flu. In addition to using the fresh leaves in your homemade juice, you can also stir in a few drops of peppermint oil.

Rosemary

Rosemary is known for its strong aroma, but it provides a number of significant health benefits as well. For example, rosemary extract helps prevent carcinogens from binding with DNA when they enter the body, thus helping reduce tumor formation. Rosemary has also been shown to stimulate the immune system, to improve digestion, and to increase blood circulation.

Sage

Sage has a lightly sweet yet savory flavor that works incredibly well in savory juice recipes. It's very rich in vitamin K, and also contains flavonoids, which have anti-inflammatory, antimicrobial, and anti-cancer properties. Sage has also been linked to increased cognitive function.

St. John's Wort

You may have never heard of St. John's wort, but after you try it, it may become a staple in your pantry. St. John's wort has been shown to help relieve mild to moderate anxiety and depression, all without the side effects that can be caused by antidepressant medications. This herb also contains melatonin, a hormone that regulates the body's sleep cycle and which may help improve the quality of your sleep.

Thyme

Thyme has a unique fragrance and is an excellent source of vitamin K. It has long been used as a natural remedy for respiratory illnesses, including coughs, bronchitis, and chest congestion. More recently, however, studies have shown that it may also provide antioxidant, antibacterial, and antimicrobial benefits. Thyme is also very nutrient dense; it's a good source of iron, manganese, calcium, and dietary fiber.

Ways Herbs Can Be Used in Juice

There are several ways to go about using herbs in fresh juice. For herbs that can be used fresh (e.g., basil, cilantro, etc.) you can simply juice the leaves and stems the same way you would other vegetables. Other herbs, however, are more difficult to come by in their fresh form. For these herbs, it may be easier to use the herb in its dried form or in a decoction. To create your own herbal decoctions, simply steep about one teaspoon of the dried herb in about one-fourth cup of water for ten minutes. After the ten minutes are up, strain the mixture to separate out the solids. Stir the liquid into one cup of fresh juice and enjoy!

If you prefer using fresh herbs in your juices, there are a few things you can do to make it easier. Unless you plan to use a whole bunch of cilantro or some other herb, it can be tricky to feed just a few sprigs through your juicer. In some cases, you may be able to wrap the sprigs around a more solid vegetable such as a carrot or stalk of celery. If this doesn't work, however, you can always try rolling the herbs into a ball and feeding it through the juicer along with the other ingredients. By forming the herbs into a ball, the mass will be more substantial so other ingredients can help push it through the feed spout.

Another option for using herbs in fresh juice is to purchase tinctures. A tincture is a liquid extract of a plant, typically made with ethanol or some other solvent like vinegar or glycerol. The benefit of tinctures over fresh herbs is that they have a much longer shelf life. They can easily be added to fresh juice, smoothies, or tea, or can even be taken directly. Make sure to follow the dosage instructions on the bottle of purchased tinctures because they come in varying strengths. If you don't want to affect the flavor of your juice but want to enhance its nutritional benefits, try adding just a few drops at a time.

Using Fresh Spices in Raw Juice

Looking to spice up your juice blend? Here's some information on the best spices to try.

- Cardamom
- Cayenne
- Chinese five-spice powder
- Cinnamon
- Cumin
- Curry

- Garlic
- Ginger
- Nutmeg
- Pumpkin pie spice
- Tarragon
- Turmeric

Cardamom

Cardamom is widely used in India. Common in Ayurvedic medicine, it's used as a treatment for digestive issues, mouth ulcers, and even depression. Cardamom has a citrusy, peppery flavor and is known for having a variety of medicinal benefits. It's been shown to help detoxify the body, to improve oral health, to relieve the symptoms of colds and the flu, and to lower blood pressure.

Cayenne

It may seem like a strange ingredient to add to raw juice, but cayenne pepper is known for its health benefits as well as its spicy flavor. Cayenne is derived from a pepper that belongs to the *Capsicum* family of vegetables, also known as chili peppers. These peppers contain high levels of vitamin A, which is essential for healthy tissue. The spicy flavor of cayenne pepper is due to high levels of capsaicin, a substance that has also been linked to pain reduction and congestion relief.

Chinese Five-Spice Powder

This spice mixture is commonly used in Chinese cuisine and contains star anise, cloves, Chinese cinnamon, Sichuan pepper, and fennel seeds. Typically used to flavor meats, it can also be added to fresh juices for a boost of flavor. All of the spices in this mixture are known for their healing properties, which makes this blend the perfect addition to healthful raw juices.

Cinnamon

Not only does cinnamon add a unique flavor to raw juice, it may also help reduce blood sugar levels. A study conducted in Germany revealed that daily consumption of cinnamon extract helped reduce blood sugar by about 10 percent. It may also help reduce cholesterol and triglycerides. To maximize the benefits of this spice, use a 1-gram capsule of cinnamon extract in juice daily.

Cumin

The spice commonly known as cumin is derived from cumin seeds ground into a powder. The powder has a nutty, peppery flavor that is popular for use in Mexican, Indian, and Middle Eastern cuisine. Cumin seed is an excellent source of iron, which is essential for healthy immune function and for the metabolism of energy. Cumin has also been linked to improved digestion and cancer prevention. Add the seeds themselves to your raw juice or stir in a little of the fresh-ground powder.

Curry

Curry is most commonly seen as a spice mixture for use in cooking, but the dried leaves of the curry plant are incredibly beneficial. These leaves are rich in a number of vitamins and minerals, including phosphorus, calcium, and iron. Curry leaves also contain valuable fibers and proteins. In terms of its medicinal benefits, curry has been linked to relief from digestive problems, skin problems, and diabetes.

Garlic

Consumption of garlic has been linked to reduced risk for ovarian, colorectal, and other types of cancer. These claims are supported by the results of several studies, including a clinical trial conducted in Japan in 2006 to test the efficacy of garlic in reducing the size and number of precancerous growths. Garlic contains almost eighty different phytochemicals, including allicin, which has been shown to decrease high blood pressure.

Ginger

Though ginger has been associated with a number of benefits, it's best known for its anti-nausea properties. This spice has been known to relieve stomach upset caused by a number of factors, including pregnancy, chemotherapy, and motion sickness. Ginger has this effect because it contains a powerful antioxidant that blocks the effects of serotonin, a chemical your brain and stomach produce when you're nauseated. Ginger also helps stop the production of free radicals, which can also contribute to nausea. Other benefits associated with ginger include decreased blood pressure, reduced cancer risk, and relief from arthritis pain.

Nutmeg

Though known primarily for its use in baked goods, nutmeg also provides a number of health benefits. For example, in ancient Greece and Rome it was used as a brain tonic to help eliminate stress and fatigue. Nutmeg has also been shown to help relieve indigestion, to improve bad breath, and to enhance relaxation to encourage sleep.

Pumpkin Pie Spice

Pumpkin pie spice is a mixture of cinnamon, ginger, nutmeg, allspice, and cloves. Typically used for seasoning pumpkin pie and other baked goods, this blend can also be used in fresh juices to give them a sweet and savory flavor. Its ingredients are known for their healing properties, which makes it a very healthful additive for fresh juice.

Tarragon

Also known as dragon wort, tarragon is often associated with Mediterranean cuisine. It's rich in phytonutrients and antioxidants, and is known for its disease-prevention properties. Another benefit of tarragon is that it contains polyphenolic compounds, which help regulate blood sugar levels. Tarragon is a good source of vitamins and minerals, including vitamins A and C, calcium, iron, and manganese. When infused in a tea, tarragon has been shown to help cure insomnia.

Turmeric

Turmeric is often used in curries and contains a powerful anti-inflammatory called curcumin. Curcumin works in a similar way to COX-2 inhibitors, a group of drugs that help to reduce the COX-2 enzymes in the body responsible for the pain and swelling of arthritis. Turmeric may also help prevent colon cancer and Alzheimer's disease, according to a clinical trial conducted in 2006 by the Johns Hopkins University School of Medicine.

PART THREE
The Juicing Diet

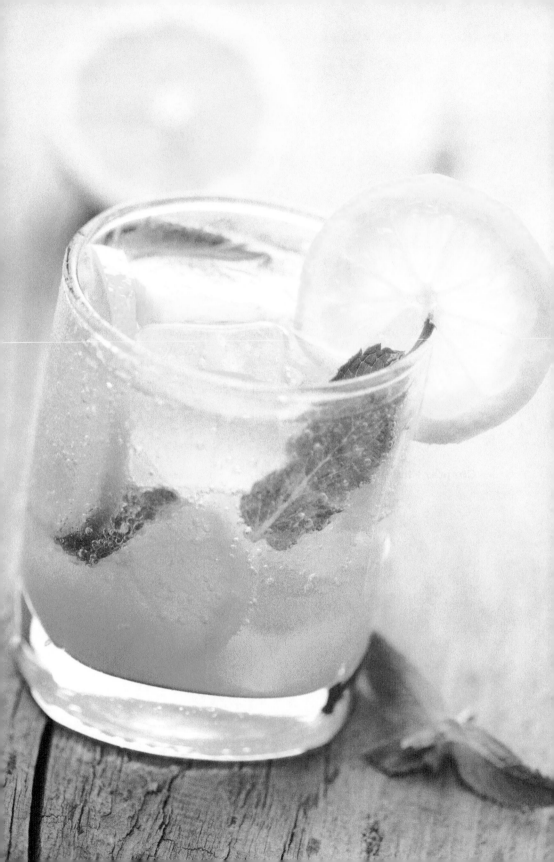

CHAPTER SIX

Juicing for Cleansing and Detox

Our bodies are naturally built to remove toxins every day as part of our normal body processes. We detox by eliminating and neutralizing toxins through our colon, liver, kidneys, lungs, lymph and skin. Detoxing through the diet is a great way to give your body a break and support its natural self-cleaning system.

—MARIA GUADAGNO, THEBOMBSHELLBLUEPRINT.COM

What Is a Juice Cleanse?

A juice cleanse is known by several different names, including juice fast and detox, and is designed to achieve a number of different goals. For some people, a juice fast is about shedding fat or retained water. It can also be a method to help combat habitual behaviors such as smoking, caffeine addiction, or overeating. Though not scientifically proven, some believe that juice fasting may even help cure chronic health problems such as depression, autoimmune diseases, and severe infections.

In layman's terms, a juice cleanse is simply a period of time during which an individual receives all of his or her daily nutrition from fruit and vegetable juices. To get the most out of a juice cleanse, these juices should be pressed at home from fresh produce or purchased from a company that produces cold-pressed juices. As you've already learned, fresh-pressed juices contain a wealth of vital nutrients that can help improve your overall health and well-being. In combination with these benefits, a juice cleanse can also help detoxify your body.

Why Is It Necessary to Detox?

Each and every day, our bodies are exposed to countless toxins through the air we breathe, the food we eat, and the substances our bodies come into contact with. Though some toxins occur naturally—mold, fungus, chemical products of metabolic processes, etc.—many are man-made. These toxins may include artificial food additives, pesticides, treated or contaminated water, processed foods, and prescription drugs. Even if you're very careful about the food you eat and the water you drink, your body is probably still being exposed to toxins you may be unaware of.

The human body is well equipped to naturally eliminate toxins, with your lungs, kidneys, liver, intestines, and skin all playing a role in detoxifying the body. Your liver is the most important organ for detoxification. It filters toxins out of your blood, allowing them to be excreted from the body through the urine. Your lungs are responsible for tackling airborne toxins, filtering them out of the air you breathe and delivering clean oxygen to other organs through your blood. Your skin also plays a significant role in detoxification, eliminating as much as one-third of the body's toxins by excreting them through your pores as you sweat.

Though your body is designed to eliminate toxins, it can handle only so many. The more toxins you take into your body (through food, liquid, and other substances), the greater your body's toxic load will be. When your toxic load becomes larger than your body can handle, excess toxins are stored in your fat cells until your body is able to deal with them. If you continue to overload your body with toxins, they will accumulate in your cells and organs, eventually leading to serious health conditions. Some of the health problems linked to toxin accumulation include:

- Feelings of sluggishness or fatigue

- Gas and bloating, particularly after meals

- Heart palpitations or failure

- Impaired vision

- Irregular or infrequent bowel movements

- Muscle aches or joint pain

- Organ dysfunction

- Skin inflammation and blemishes

A juice cleanse can be instrumental in helping your body get rid of accumulated toxins in a number of ways. Perhaps the most important way is by halting the consumption of processed foods and other toxin-laden substances. If you stop putting toxins into your body, your body will be able to tackle the toxins that have already accumulated over time. Additionally, fresh fruit and vegetable juices will provide your body with the nutrients needed to support healthy organ function as well as your body's natural detoxification processes.

Potential Side Effects

Juice cleanses are not ideal for everyone. It's a good idea to consult a doctor before making any big dietary change, especially if you have any health issues. Depending on your health and eating habits, you may experience some side effects. Mild side effects are common with any type of fast or cleanse, so don't be alarmed if you experience them yourself. If the side effects are extreme or prolonged, however, you should seek medical attention. Some side effects commonly associated with juice fasts or cleanses include:

- Diarrhea or increase in frequency of urination

- Difficulty concentrating, loss of mental clarity

- Feeling sluggish or listless, low on energy

- Headaches or irritability

- Reduced blood sugar levels—dizziness upon standing is possible

Remember, if the side effects of the juice cleanse are too much for you, you may need to take a break. The recommended duration of a juice cleanse is around three days. The longer you go, the more side effects you are likely to experience. Don't feel bad if you need to cut a seven-day juice cleanse down to three or four days. Listen to your body, and don't try to push yourself beyond your limits!

Tips for Juice Cleansing

A juice cleanse can be a great way to jump-start your journey into juicing. If you've never done one before, however, you may want to learn a few basics first. The following tips will help you to succeed in your juice cleanse or detox program.

- Always consult a physician before starting a juice cleanse. This is especially important if you have a serious medical condition like diabetes.

- Juice cleanses are not recommended for women who are pregnant or nursing.

- Buy all of the produce you need two or three days at a time. This ensures that the produce you use in your juices is fresh.

- Take advantage of seasonal produce and farmers' markets to find fresh, affordable produce.

- Drink plenty of water while cleansing to help flush toxins from your body.

- Don't engage in strenuous exercise while on a juice cleanse. If you must exercise, limit yourself to twenty to thirty minutes of mild effort.

- Include a variety of vegetables and fruits in your juice to ensure that your basic nutritional needs are met.

- Keep in mind that a juice cleanse is not a substitute for medical treatment or diagnosis.

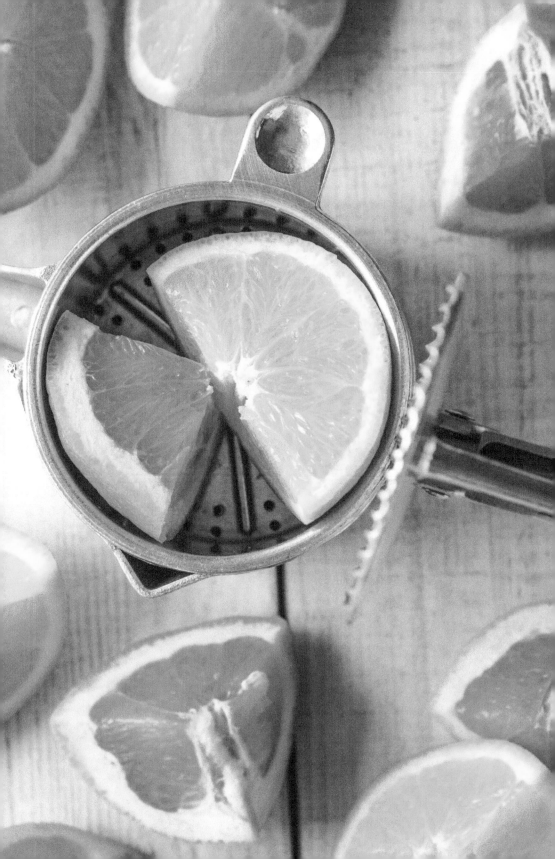

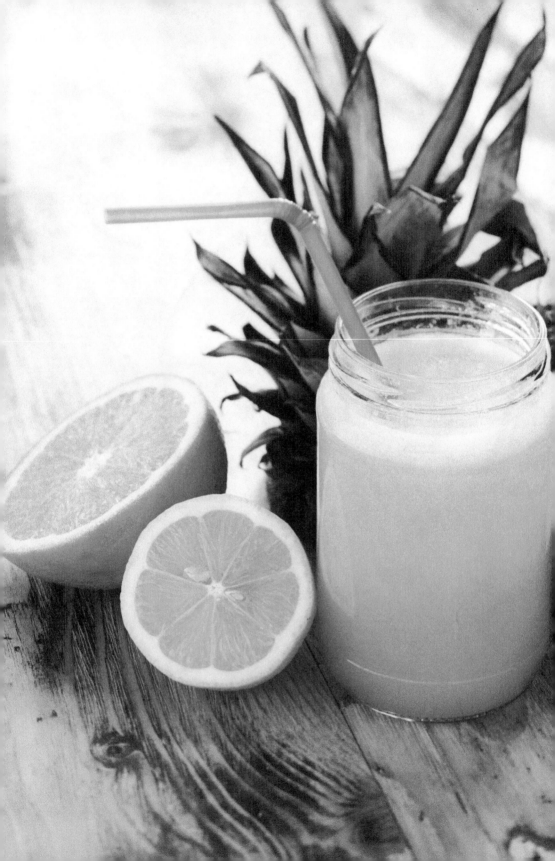

CHAPTER SEVEN

Juice as a Disease Fighter

We have scientific evidence that the right raw materials and nutritional factors can double or triple the protective power of the immune system. It is possible to hardly ever get sick, and boosting your body's defenses to the level of super immunity can save your life.

—DR. JOEL FUHRMAN, *SUPER IMMUNITY*

Though genetics and lifestyle play a role in determining how susceptible you are to certain diseases, your diet is the primary factor. The healthier your diet, the healthier your body will be overall and the better equipped it will be to fight off disease. If you pump your body full of toxins, fast food, and refined carbs, your body won't be able to function at its optimal level. Not only will this affect things like your digestion, sleep patterns, and appearance, but it can also have a significant effect on your ability to fight off disease. In this chapter you'll learn the basics of how your diet can affect your immune system, and how juicing can boost your body's disease-fighting abilities.

Diet and Its Effect on Immunity

Dr. Joel Fuhrman, author of *Super Immunity*, asks the question: "Why do some of us get sick with greater frequency than others?" As a leading expert in disease prevention, Fuhrman understands how conditions like the common cold work and, more important, how they can be stopped. Fuhrman suggests that by consuming fresh fruits and vegetables, we can supercharge our immune systems to protect our bodies from disease—everything from the common cold or flu to chronic diseases like cancer. The modern American diet is founded on unhealthful, nutrient-poor foods like processed foods and refined carbs. By changing our dietary habits, we can improve the way our bodies function and strengthen our immune systems against disease.

You probably know that a healthful diet can help prevent disease and thus lower your annual medical expenses. You may be wondering, however, what exactly constitutes a "healthful diet." There are three criteria that can be used to evaluate the quality of a diet: micronutrient content, macronutrient ratios, and avoiding toxic substances. Micronutrients are nutrients required by the human body in small quantities to maintain healthful physiological function. Some examples of micronutrients include vitamins, minerals, phytochemicals, and trace elements. Macronutrients are the nutrients the human body needs in the largest amounts, including protein, carbohydrate, and fats.

Nutrients for Immunity

A recent national conference held in Atlanta, Georgia, brought together top scientists in the fields of immunology and nutrition to discuss the correlation between diet and healthy immune system function. The goal of this conference was to discuss which nutrients are most important for immunity. It has long been known and understood that macronutrients play an essential role in supporting the body's disease-fighting abilities, but it's only recently that studies of micronutrients in relation to immune system health have been conducted. Some of the most important micronutrients for immune system health include:

Arginine: Arginine is a type of amino acid that helps improve T-cell response. This plays a role in surgical recovery and may also help with AIDS and cancer. In high quantities, arginine can compete with lysine, another amino acid beneficial in keeping viruses in check.

Vitamin A: Vitamin A, or retinol, is a fat-soluble vitamin that has been shown to improve white blood cell function. It also enhances the body's ability to resist carcinogens and infections, helping to maintain skin defenses as well.

B vitamins: B vitamins have been shown to work best together as a B complex. Certain B vitamins such as B_6 and B_{12} have been shown to slow the progression of AIDS. Deficiency in B vitamins can lead to decreased white blood cell response and shrinkage of the thymus, the organ that is critical to immune system function.

Carotenoids and beta-carotene: Beta-carotene is a powerful antioxidant that has been shown to help prevent cancer and help repair cellular damage caused by free radicals. Carotenoids like lycopene and zeaxanthin have also been shown to have anti-cancer properties.

Vitamin C: Vitamin C is one of the most well-known nutrients for immune system function. It has been shown to have both antiviral and anti-cancer properties. It has also been shown to combat inflammation. Unlike animals, humans cannot produce extra vitamin C. In times of stress, vitamin C supplementation is particularly important.

Vitamin E: Vitamin E deficiency is fairly common, and even a small daily dosage between 400 IU and 800 IU can significantly reduce your risk for infection. Too much vitamin E, however, can be immunosuppressive. Even this, however, can be useful; in the case of autoimmune conditions, vitamin E can be used to restrain overactive immune systems.

Iron: As is true of several nutrients (including vitamin E), iron is most effective in limited doses—too much can actually be dangerous. Too little iron can paralyze immune system response. This is especially true in the case of tetanus vaccines, which are only marginally effective in iron-deficient individuals.

Selenium: Selenium is particularly instrumental in the survival of AIDS patients. It has also been shown to protect the heart against viruses. Most important, selenium deficiencies have been shown to allow viruses to mutate into more dangerous forms.

Zinc: Several studies, particularly the work of Dr. Ranjit Chandra, have proven that zinc can be used to restore immunity. Limited doses of zinc are recommended, however—more than 100 milligrams per day can actually be immunosuppressive.

Juicing to Fight Disease

Now that you understand how the nutrients found in fresh fruits and vegetables can help boost the immune system, you may be wondering which fruits and vegetables are the most beneficial. Below you'll find a list of common diseases and conditions along with recommendations for fruits and vegetables best suited to fight these problems.

Allergies: Allergies are your immune system's reaction to foreign objects. These objects may be as simple as dust, pet dander, or mold, and they may bother some individuals more than others. Some of the best ingredients for juices to fight allergies include beets, carrot, celery, and pineapple. Pineapple contains an enzyme called bromelain, which helps to reduce nasal inflammation, particularly important when fighting allergies.

Asthma: Asthma is a condition that involves the constriction of the bronchioles, which can lead to restricted airways and difficulty breathing. Some causes include allergies, diet, infection, and pollution. Fruits and vegetables recommended to support the management of asthma are apples, carrots, celery, citrus, cucumber, peppermint, and turnip.

Cold, flu, and fever: Though there is no cure for the common cold, certain nutrients can help your body fight off the virus. Carrots, lemons, and oranges are all excellent sources of vitamin C, which helps improve your body's ability to fight infection. Garlic is also beneficial for treating colds because it's a natural antibiotic.

Colitis: Colitis is a condition affecting the digestive system, similar to Crohn's disease and irritable bowel syndrome (IBS). The condition involves inflammation of the bowel and may be the result of infection or autoimmune reaction. Some of the ingredients recommended for colitis include aloe vera, bananas, cantaloupe, melon, nectarines, and wheatgrass.

Crohn's disease: This is an autoimmune disorder that results in inflammation and ulceration in the digestive tract. Stress is thought to be a trigger, and abnormal immune reactions to bacteria may also play a role. Some of the ingredients recommended for this condition include aloe vera, cabbage, cantaloupe, carrots, celery, and nectarines.

Diabetes: Diabetes is a chronic condition that is becoming increasingly prevalent in the United States. The condition is linked to high blood sugar levels and can be exacerbated by the consumption of high-glycemic foods. Vegetable like Brussels sprouts and string beans are beneficial for diabetics because they act as a mild diuretic, helping to flush toxins from the body.

Heart disease: One of the major factors in determining your risk for heart disease is blood pressure. Beets are known to be particularly beneficial in helping to lower and regulate blood pressure levels. This is due to their high concentration of heart-healthful compounds such as vitamins C and K, fiber, polyphenols, and nitrates.

Rheumatoid arthritis: This condition results in pain and inflammation around the bones, muscles, and joints. Though genetic factors play a key role in determining your risk for this disease, overconsumption of dairy can also play a role. Some of the best ingredients for fighting this disease include blackberries, cabbage, cherries, mint, spring greens, watermelon, and zucchini.

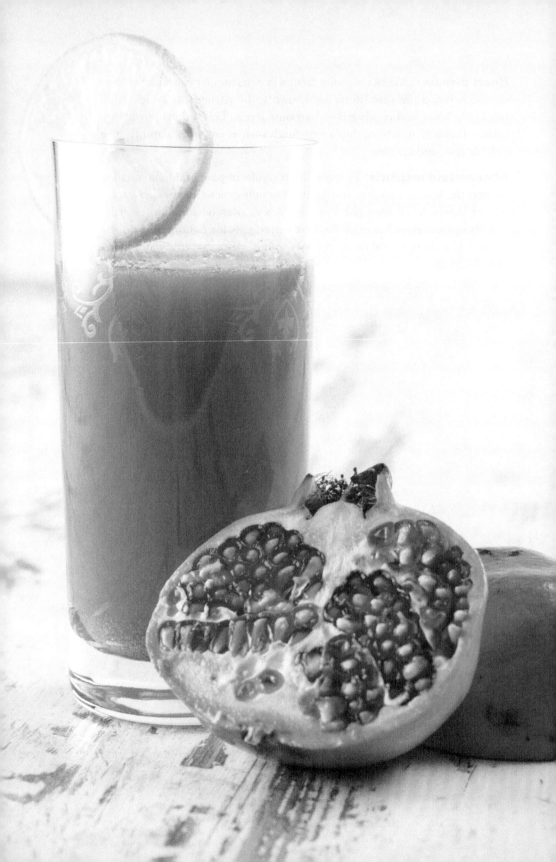

CHAPTER EIGHT

Juicing for Beauty

Skin conditions often occur because skin is our largest eliminative organ. When our body cannot rid of toxins and is not flowing properly, it forces out impurities through the skin, causing many different types of conditions. Juice fasts and detox programs have shown to have a great effect for those with skin problems.

—VANESSA SIMKINS, *THE JUICING MIXOLOGIST*

Causes of Common Skin Problems

Skin problems are fairly common, and medications or topical ointments are often the treatment of choice. But you may be surprised to hear that juicing can actually help naturally resolve or even reverse some skin conditions. Before we get into that, however, you should take a few minutes to learn the causes behind some of the most common skin problems.

Aging: As you age, your skin will naturally go through some changes. Not only will you develop wrinkles but your skin may lose some of its hydration and elasticity, causing it to sag in places.

Improper pH balance: Your skin has a natural pH of around 5.5, which makes it slightly acidic. Skin products, including soap, can increase the pH of your skin dramatically, causing it to become very alkaline. The more alkaline your skin gets, the drier and more sensitive it will become, sometimes resulting in problems like eczema or inflammation.

Poor nutrition: If you do not provide your body with the nutrients it needs to maintain proper function, you cannot expect it to be healthy. This goes for your skin as well as your organs.

Smoking: Smoking causes a variety of health problems, including damage to your skin. Studies have shown that smokers tend to have more wrinkles than nonsmokers, regardless of age, complexion, and sun exposure.

Stress: Though you may not realize it, stress plays a role in nearly all of your body's systems and functions. When your body is under stress, it releases hormones, including cortisol and adrenaline, both of which can have an adverse effect on your skin. Cortisol production leads to an increase in blood sugar levels, which can damage the collagen in your skin. Adrenaline shifts blood flow away from your skin toward more vital functions, which can dull your complexion due to oxygen loss.

Sun damage: You probably already know that exposure to ultraviolet (UV) rays can damage your skin. This type of light damages elastin fibers in the skin, which can lead to a loss of elasticity. Sun-damaged skin may also bruise easily and can take longer to heal.

Toxicity: In the last chapter you learned about some of the dangers of processed foods and how they can lead to toxicity in the body. You also learned that the skin plays an important role in removing these toxins. It makes sense, then, that the more toxins your skin is responsible for eliminating, the more stress it will be under. Increased toxic loads can result in a variety of skin conditions.

Juicing to Improve Skin Health

A study conducted by German scientists at the Institute for Experimental Dermatology revealed that increased consumption of fruits and vegetables had a positive effect on skin condition. Not only did it help to clear up blemishes but it also increased the thickness and hydration of skin. All in all, twenty-six middle-aged female participants experienced a 39 percent increase in microcirculation of the skin, with 9 percent more hydration and a 16 percent increase in skin density. As the study shows, the phytonutrients and antioxidants found in fresh fruits and vegetables help improve skin metabolism, which has a positive effect on the hydration, thickness, and density of skin. Notably, the fruits and vegetables consumed by participants in the study were in juice form.

This study is just one of many that points toward a connection between juicing and improved skin. Some of the fruit and vegetable ingredients most beneficial for skin health include:

- Apple
- Artichoke
- Avocado
- Banana
- Beets (and beet greens)
- Blueberries
- Broccoli
- Carrots
- Coconut
- Cucumber
- Dandelion greens
- Fennel
- Flaxseed
- Garlic
- Kale
- Kiwi
- Mango
- Nuts
- Papaya
- Pineapple
- Pomegranate
- Pumpkin
- Tomato

Including some of these fruits and vegetables in your juicing regimen can help relieve a variety of skin problems. The essential fatty acids found in avocado, raw nuts, and seeds can help alleviate dry skin. These foods may also help relieve inflammatory conditions like rosacea and even serious skin conditions like psoriasis. To get the most benefit for skin health out of your juices, combine them with detoxifying ingredients like those mentioned previously.

Juicing Benefits for Antiaging

By now you're probably a believer in the healing power of fresh fruits and vegetables. You may be skeptical, however, to hear that juicing can actually *reverse* some of the effects of aging. Before you can understand how juicing may provide antiaging benefits, you need to understand the aging process itself. Symptoms of aging such as wrinkles, dryness, and decreased elasticity of skin are the result of cell death. From the minute you're born, your cells begin to die at a rate as fast as one billion cells per minute. Luckily, the human body produces plenty of new cells, so the loss of these dead cells is not a problem. As you get older, however, the rate of cell regeneration starts to slow down so your cells start to die more quickly than they can be replaced, resulting in the appearance of aging.

Though you cannot stop your body from aging, you can mitigate the symptoms of aging, particularly those symptoms that affect your physical appearance. One of the main causes of premature aging is toxicity. The larger your body's toxic load, the more your skin will succumb to the symptoms of aging. Cleansing your body by reducing your intake of toxins and increasing your intake of vital nutrients will help slow the rate of cell death, enabling your skin to maintain its youthful appearance. As you have already learned, juicing can play an important role in detoxifying the body. The results of a detox or juice cleanse will be evident in the improved health of your skin, hair, and nails.

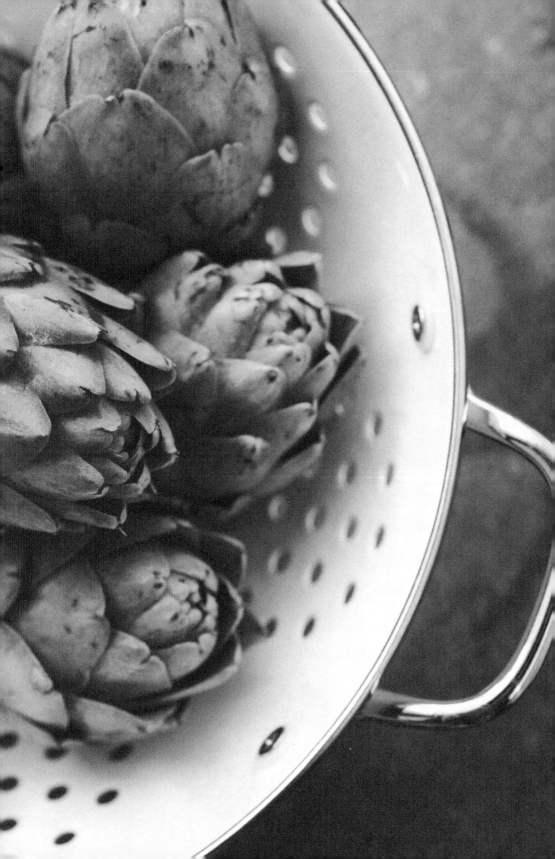

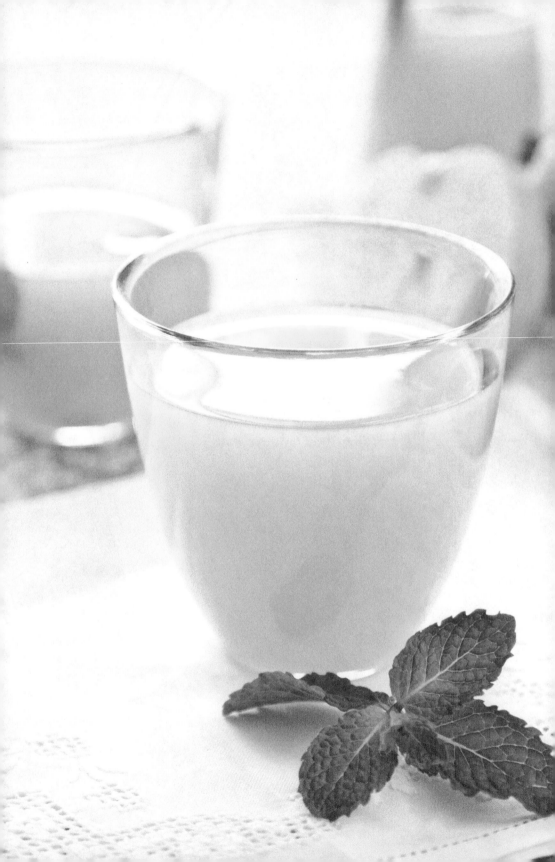

CHAPTER NINE

Juicing for Weight Loss

A recent study...showed amazing health benefits from choosing raw foods—freshly made juice is the supreme raw food. The study showed that more than 80 percent of the people surveyed lost weight. But that was only the beginning of their transformation.

—LINDA WAGNER, *JUICE FEASTING 101*

One of the main reasons people turn to juicing is to lose weight. Though juicing can be a healthful addition to any weight-loss program, it's not a guaranteed way to lose weight in and of itself. A healthful weight-loss plan involves a number of factors: healthful eating habits, reduced calorie intake, exercise, and willpower. As long as you look at juicing as a tool for achieving your weight-loss goals and not a cure-all solution, you'll be delighted by the ways juicing can help transform your life and your body.

How Juicing for Weight Loss Works

Adding a glass of freshly pressed juice to your daily dietary intake is not a guaranteed way to lose weight. If you make some positive changes to your dietary habits, however, in addition to incorporating fresh juices into your diet, then you'll be pleasantly surprised at the results. Many people struggle to lose weight following one fad diet after another. You may lose weight at first, but eventually your weight loss will plateau or reverse itself entirely. Juicing is a key component in an overall healthful lifestyle that will not only help you lose weight but keep it off for good.

Juicing helps promote weight loss in a variety of ways. First, by replacing one or two unhealthful meals or snacks per day with a glass of fresh juice, you can significantly lower your daily caloric intake. As you surely already know, the only way to lose weight is to take in fewer calories than you burn. In addition to moderate exercise several times a week, replacing unhealthful food choices with fresh juice will help kick-start your weight-loss efforts.

Juicing may also help cleanse your body of accumulated toxins in your fat cells that contribute to significant health problems such as liver dysfunction and obesity. Freshly pressed juices contain key nutrients needed to flush those accumulated toxins from your body, thereby restoring healthy function

FAST-FOOD BEVERAGES VERSUS FRESH JUICE

	MCDONALD'S BLUEBERRY POMEGRANATE SMOOTHIE	BASKIN ROBBINS' MANGO FRUIT BLAST	BURGER KING'S MOCHA FRAPPÉ	FRESH KALE, BROCCOLI, AND APPLE JUICE
Serving size	12 oz	12 oz	16 oz	12 oz
Calories	220	250	510	184
Calories from fat	5	5	200	5
Fat	1 g	1 g	22 g	1 g
Carbs	50 g	61 g	72 g	42 g
Protein	2 g	1 g	4 g	6 g
Fiber	3 g	1 g	0 g	9 g
Sugar	44 g	60 g	49 g	21 g

to your organs. The more efficiently your body operates, the more it can utilize nutrients for fuel instead of storing them as fat.

View the Fast-Food Beverages versus Fresh Juice table to compare the nutrition facts of several popular fast-food beverages to the same kale, broccoli, and apple juice mentioned earlier in this book.

Looking at the table, you may notice several things. First, the calorie counts of the fast-food beverages are significantly higher than that of the fresh juice in all three cases, even when taking into account the larger serving size of the frappé. You may also notice that, despite being the same size or smaller than the fast-food beverages, the fresh juice has a higher content of both protein and fiber. The most striking difference between the fresh juice and the fast-food beverages, however, is the sugar content. The fresh juice contains 21 grams of sugar, but all of that sugar is in the form of natural, simple sugars that are easily absorbed by the body as an energy source. The McDonald's Blueberry Pomegranate Smoothie has more than double the amount of sugar, much of it added.

Based on the table's information, it should be obvious to you that fresh homemade juice is significantly more nutritious than fast-food beverages. You may feel like you are making a healthful choice in ordering a smoothie or coffee to go with your meal over a soft drink or milkshake, but that may not actually be true. The first step in achieving your weight-loss goals is to pay greater attention to the amount and types of food you put into your body. By fueling your body with healthful, nutrient-rich foods rather than high-calorie, unhealthful foods, you can improve your health and achieve your weight-loss goals.

Weight-Loss Tips for Juicing

Juicing is not a miracle prescription for weight loss, but it is a key component of a healthful lifestyle—the type of lifestyle that supports healthful weight loss and maintenance of that weight loss. Keep the following tips in mind as you incorporate juicing into your weight-loss efforts:

- Start off slowly by replacing one meal a day with fresh-pressed juice. The best meal to start with is breakfast, because fresh juice will provide your body with the nutrients it needs to start your day off right.

- Be mindful of how much juice you are consuming. Even though it's much lower in calories than sugary beverages, you should be careful about adding too much juice to your diet without making other dietary adjustments.

- Don't try to lose weight too quickly by severely reducing your caloric intake. Weight that is lost quickly is regained quickly once you resume your regular dietary habits.

- Try to incorporate other healthful eating habits into your life in addition to juicing. Swap high-calorie snacks for a salad or a piece of fruit.

- Make sure to work thirty minutes of moderate exercise into your day at least three times a week. Regular exercise will not only ramp up your weight loss but will also improve cardiovascular function and improve your energy levels and sense of overall well-being.

- Don't be afraid to experiment with different flavors. Try combining both fruits and vegetables to create sweet-tasting beverages.

- Take advantage of local farmers' markets and health food stores for fresh seasonal produce.

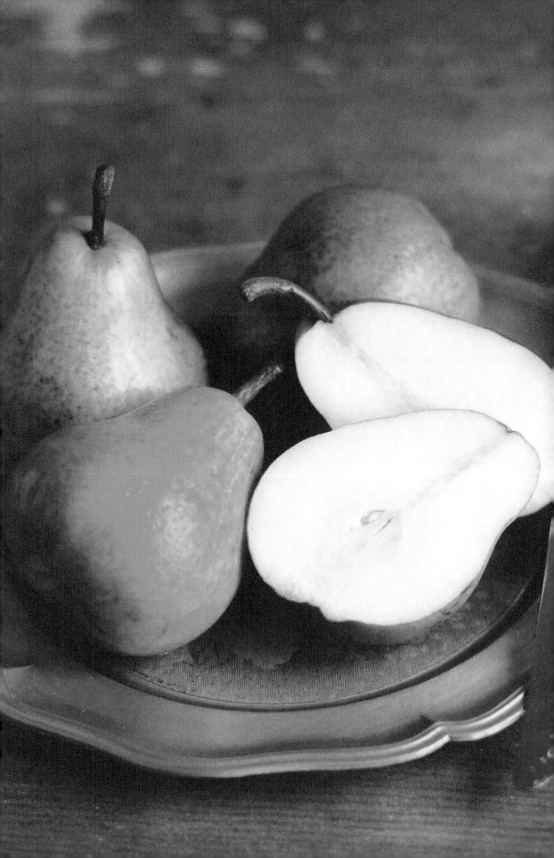

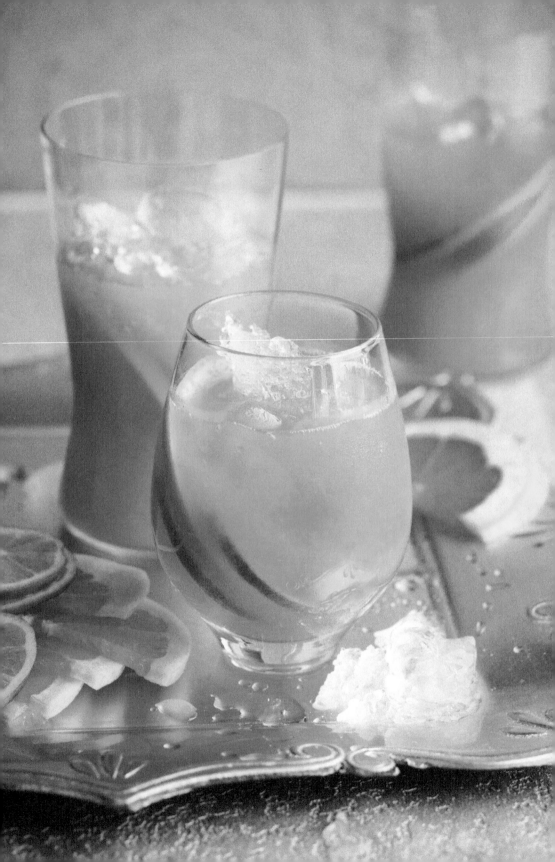

CHAPTER TEN

30-Day Juicing Weight-Loss Plan

More and more celebrities, athletes and people of all ages and walks of life are turning to juicing and green smoothies to lose weight and improve their overall health. Why? Because they have found that juicing is changing their lives—giving them more energy, better sleep, stronger immune systems, brighter skin and a younger appearance.

—CHERIE CALBOM, *THE JUICE LADY'S BIG BOOK OF JUICES AND GREEN SMOOTHIES*

Engaging in thirty straight days of juicing is not practical for most people for a variety of reasons. For many people, side effects such as headaches and sluggishness settle in after a few days on a liquid diet, which can get in the way of a full-time job or busy life. Other people simply don't want to give up solid food for such a long period of time. The following thirty-day plan combines the benefits of juicing and eating healthful, solid foods to help you achieve your weight-loss goals.

7-Day Diet Reboot Plan

To get the most out of your juicing weight-loss plan, you need to take some time to eliminate the unhealthful foods from your diet. Follow the guidelines below over a seven-day period to prepare for your juice cleanse.

Day 1: Reduce the amount of refined carbs and fast food you eat. This includes white flour, sugar, and other junk foods.

Day 2: Eliminate processed meats from your diet, like bacon and deli meats.

Day 3: Reduce your intake of caffeine. Try to eliminate it completely over the next few days.

Day 4: Begin to drink one to two glasses of fruit and/or vegetable juice a day. Work these in for breakfast or snacks.

Day 5: Start to incorporate more fresh fruits and vegetables into your diet, including salads, whole fruits, nuts, and seeds.

Day 6: Eliminate meat from your diet completely, replacing it with additional vegetables and fruits.

Day 7: Eliminate dairy from your diet. This includes milk, cheese, yogurt, and ice cream.

5-Day Juicing for Weight Loss Intro

This intro is designed to get you into the habit of eating only fruits and vegetables for an extended period of time. During these first five days, you will still eat three meals per day, supplementing them with fresh-pressed juices as snacks in between each meal. You'll find recipes for all the juices listed later in this book. The following meal plans are only a suggestion—feel free to find recipes for your own healthful salads, soups, and side dishes.

Day 8

Drink 8 to 12 ounces hot lemon water upon waking.
Breakfast: Cinnamon apple granola
Snack: Spinach Basil Lime Juice
Lunch: Strawberry kale salad
Snack: Ruby-Red Juice Blend
Dinner: Vegan stuffed peppers

Day 9

Drink 8 to 12 ounces hot lemon water upon waking.
Breakfast: Tomato basil omelet
Snack: Lemongrass Apple Juice
Lunch: Butternut squash soup
Snack: Broccoli Beet Blast
Dinner: Baked vegetable casserole

Day 10

Drink 8 to 12 ounces hot lemon water upon waking.
Breakfast: Eggs scrambled with tomato and scallions
Snack: Take Charge Turnip Booster
Lunch: Sweet apple spinach salad
Snack: Green Dream Juice Blend
Dinner: Winter vegetable stew

Day 11

Drink 8 to 12 ounces hot lemon water upon waking.
Breakfast: Maple walnut granola
Snack: Savory Spring Green Juice
Lunch: Tomato basil bisque
Snack: Triple Berry Tonic
Dinner: Roasted rosemary vegetables

Day 12

Drink 8 to 12 ounces hot lemon water upon waking.
Breakfast: Spinach and onion omelet
Snack: Ginger Vegetable Juice Blend
Lunch: Spring green and scallions salad
Snack: Honeyed Cantaloupe Tonic
Dinner: Vegan eggplant Parmesan

15-Day Juice Cleanse

After making the effort to clean up your eating habits, you are now ready to engage in a fifteen-day juice cleanse. Below you'll find recommendations for five juices to drink each day for a total of fifteen days. Be sure to follow the juicing tips provided throughout the book and take into account the information from the Juicing for Weight Loss chapter as well. In addition to three "meal" juices per day, you are allowed two "snack" juices. Feel free to choose recipes from this book or create your own juicing combinations. Limit your snack juices to 8 ounces and your meal juices to 12 to 16 ounces.

Day 13

Breakfast: Rousing Raspberry Radish Juice
Snack: 8 ounces green juice
Lunch: Pretty in Pink
Snack: 8 ounces green juice
Dinner: Cayenne Red Pepper Juice Blend

Day 14

Breakfast: Tropical Sunrise Green Juice
Snack: 8 ounces green juice
Lunch: Minty Melon Juice Blend
Snack: 8 ounces green juice
Dinner: Green Bean Sprout Power Juice

Day 15

Breakfast: Green Machine Juice Booster
Snack: 8 ounces green juice
Lunch: Easy Breeze Blueberry Blend
Snack: 8 ounces green juice
Dinner: Zesty Zucchini Juice

Day 16

Breakfast: Berry Basil Blusher
Snack: 8 ounces green juice
Lunch: Groovy Green Juice
Snack: 8 ounces green juice
Dinner: Curried Juice Cocktail

Day 17

Breakfast: On-the-Go Morning Booster
Snack: 8 ounces green juice
Lunch: Fruity Fennel Juice Blend

Snack: 8 ounces green juice
Dinner: Cabbage Wheatgrass Tonic

Day 18

Breakfast: Kiwi Lime Spritzer
Snack: 8 ounces green juice
Lunch: Garden Greens Juice Blend
Snack: 8 ounces green juice
Dinner: Tomato and Spinach Juice

Day 19

Breakfast: Lemongrass Apple Juice
Snack: 8 ounces green juice
Lunch: Get Your Greens Here
Snack: 8 ounces green juice
Dinner: Red-Hot V-6 Juice

Day 20

Breakfast: Wonderful Weight-Loss Juice
Snack: 8 ounces green juice
Lunch: Papaya Nectarine Juice
Snack: 8 ounces green juice
Dinner: Red and Green Radish Juice

Day 21

Breakfast: Just Plain Green Juice
Snack: 8 ounces green juice
Lunch: Sweet Pea Power-Up Juice
Snack: 8 ounces green juice
Dinner: Lean Mean Green Juice Blend

Day 22

Breakfast: Get Your Juices Flowing
Snack: 8 ounces green juice
Lunch: Black Cherry Basil Blast
Snack: 8 ounces green juice
Dinner: Cleansing Cauliflower Carrot Juice

Day 23

Breakfast: Pomegranate Pleasure
Snack: 8 ounces green juice
Lunch: Spinach Cucumber Celery Juice
Snack: 8 ounces green juice
Dinner: Cranberry Rhubarb Cooler

Day 24

Breakfast: Brilliant Blueberry Breakfast Blend
Snack: 8 ounces green juice
Lunch: Peachy Parsley Juice
Snack: 8 ounces green juice
Dinner: Indian-Style Green Mango Juice

Day 25

Breakfast: Kale Cabbage Juice
Snack: 8 ounces green juice
Lunch: Iced Pear Juice
Snack: 8 ounces green juice
Dinner: Avocado Asparagus Juice

Day 26

Breakfast: Sunrise Citrus Spritzer
Snack: 8 ounces green juice
Lunch: Cilantro Coconut Chiller
Snack: 8 ounces green juice
Dinner: Tart and Tangy Tomato Juice

Day 27

Breakfast: Razzy Rainbow Juice
Snack: 8 ounces green juice
Lunch: Blueberry Banana Booster
Snack: 8 ounces green juice
Dinner: Basil Ginger Juice Blend

3-Day Healthful Diet Transition

Now that you've completed your fifteen-day juice cleanse you are ready to start transitioning back into a "normal" diet. Take the healthful habits you've learned throughout this weight-loss plan and continue to implement them in your daily life. Over the next three days, slowly begin to work solid food back into your diet in the form of salads, soups, and cooked vegetables.

Day 28

Breakfast: Fruit-based juice
Snack: Vegetable-based juice
Lunch: Fresh vegetable salad with fruit
Snack: Green juice
Dinner: Sweet or savory juice

Day 29

Breakfast: Green juice
Snack: Vegetable-based juice
Lunch: Fresh vegetable salad with fruit
Snack: Fruit-based juice
Dinner: Fresh vegetable soup

Day 30

Breakfast: Fresh vegetable omelet
Snack: Green juice
Lunch: Fresh vegetable salad with fruit
Snack: Fruit-based juice
Dinner: Roasted mixed vegetables

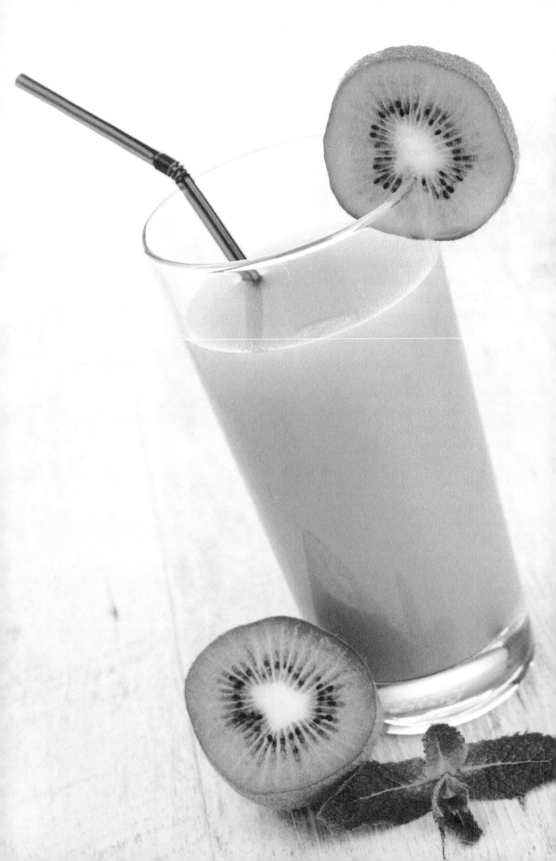

CHAPTER ELEVEN

Health Checklist
What Juice Is Best for You?

If you're struggling with your health, there is hope for you, no matter what challenges you face. Never, ever give up. There's a purpose for your life. You need to be healthy and strong to complete your purpose. To that end, [juicing] can help you live your life to the fullest.

—CHERIE CALBOM, *THE JUICE LADY'S BIG BOOK OF JUICES AND GREEN SMOOTHIES*

When it comes to preparing your own homemade juices, the possibilities are endless. In this book alone you'll find recipes that include more than seventy different ingredients! After reading the last few chapters, you should understand the significant benefits that fruits and vegetables can provide for certain diseases and conditions. If you're looking for a recipe that will provide specific benefits, you're in the right place. The following chart outlines the key benefits of the majority of the fruits and vegetables used in the recipes included in this book. Using this chart, you can create your own juicing combinations to provide the particular benefits you're looking for. You can also use this chart to pick out recipes that contain the right ingredients.

BENEFITS OF JUICING INGREDIENTS

INGREDIENT	ENERGY	ANTI-CANCER	DETOX	HEART HEALTH	IMMUNE HEALTH	BONE HEALTH	DIGES-TION	SKIN BEAUTY	BRAIN HEALTH
Apple		x	x						x
Apricot					x			x	
Arugula		x				x	x		
Asparagus	x	x				x	x	x	x
Beets		x				x			x
Bell pepper		x			x	x		x	
Blackberry			x			x	x		
Blood orange			x	x		x		x	
Blueberries			x			x	x		
Bok choy		x		x		x		x	x
Broccoli	x	x				x	x	x	
Brussels sprouts		x	x				x		
Cabbage			x			x			x
Cantaloupe		x		x	x	x			x
Carrots		x		x	x	x		x	
Cauliflower			x			x			x
Celeriac		x			x	x	x		x
Celery		x	x			x			
Cherries		x				x			x
Cilantro				x		x			x
Collard greens	x	x		x		x		x	
Cranberries		x		x	x		x		

BENEFITS OF JUICING INGREDIENTS

INGREDIENT	ENERGY	ANTI-CANCER	DETOX	HEART HEALTH	IMMUNE HEALTH	BONE HEALTH	DIGES-TION	SKIN BEAUTY	BRAIN HEALTH
Dandelion greens	X	X	X			X	X	X	
Figs		X		X		X			
Garlic		X		X					X
Ginger			X				X		X
Gooseberries		X		X	X	X			X
Grapes		X	X						X
Grapefruit		X	X	X		X		X	
Guava						X		X	
Honeydew		X		X					X
Jicama				X	X		X	X	
Kale		X		X		X			
Kiwi	X		X			X	X	X	
Kohlrabi	X	X		X				X	
Kumquat			X	X		X		X	
Lemon		X	X				X		
Lime		X	X				X		
Mango		X		X	X		X	X	
Mint		X		X			X		
Mustard greens	X	X					X	X	
Nectarine			X	X		X		X	
Onion		X				X			X
Orange			X	X		X		X	

BENEFITS OF JUICING INGREDIENTS

INGREDIENT	ENERGY	ANTI-CANCER	DETOX	HEART HEALTH	IMMUNE HEALTH	BONE HEALTH	DIGES-TION	SKIN BEAUTY	BRAIN HEALTH
Papaya		X		X	X	X	X	X	X
Parsley		X	X	X					
Parsnip		X	X			X			
Passion fruit				X			X		X
Peach		X		X	X			X	X
Pear			X			X	X		
Peas	X			X		X	X		
Persimmon		X			X				
Pineapple			X	X		X			
Plum		X			X		X		
Pome-granate		X	X						X
Pumpkin		X		X	X	X		X	
Radish		X	X				X		
Raspberries		X		X		X		X	
Romaine letuce	X	X		X		X	X	X	
Rutabaga		X		X		X	X		
Scallions		X		X	X	X			
Spinach	X	X				X	X	X	X
Starfruit				X	X	X			
Straw-berries		X		X					X
Summer squash		X		X					X

BENEFITS OF JUICING INGREDIENTS

INGREDIENT	ENERGY	ANTI-CANCER	DETOX	HEART HEALTH	IMMUNE HEALTH	BONE HEALTH	DIGES-TION	SKIN BEAUTY	BRAIN HEALTH
Sweet potato		x	x		x		x	x	
Swiss chard	x	x		x		x	x	x	
Tangerine		x	x	x					
Tomato		x		x		x		x	x
Turnips		x	x	x			x		
Turnip greens	x	x				x		x	
Water-melon		x		x		x			
Wheatgrass	x		x		x	x	x	x	
Zucchini		x		x		x			

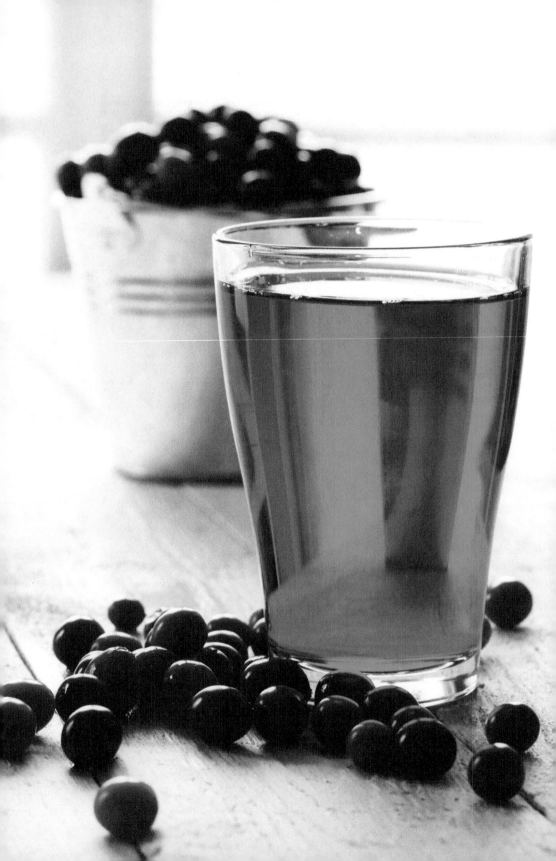

CHAPTER TWELVE

10 Steps for Success

It's natural for anyone trying to lose weight to want to lose it very quickly. But evidence shows that people who lose weight gradually and steadily (about 1 to 2 lbs. per week) are more successful at keeping weight off. Losing weight is not easy and it takes commitment.

—CENTERS FOR DISEASE CONTROL AND PREVENTION

By now you know just how beneficial juicing can be for your overall health. Before you dive in, however, you may want to take some of these tips into consideration.

1. **Choose the right juicer.** If you plan to make juicing a part of your daily routine, you'll need to invest in a high-quality juicer that will stand up to frequent use. You should also think carefully about the pros and cons of each model and which one would best suit you and your family.

2. **Use a grocery list.** Before going to the store to buy supplies for juicing, prepare a grocery list. Fresh produce—especially if you decide to go organic—can be expensive. Without a plan, you may end up walking out with a fuller cart (and emptier wallet) than you expected.

3. **Prepare your ingredients correctly.** Make sure to wash all of your produce before you use it to get rid of dirt and pesticide residues.

You may even want to rinse and prepare all of your produce when you get home from the store so it's ready to use when you need it.

4. **Clean your juicer immediately after each use.** Some juicers are trickier to clean than others, but the same can be said for every model: the sooner you clean it after using it, the easier your job will be. Don't wait for pulp to dry and stick to the sides of your juicer's grater basket. Rinse it immediately and save yourself the headache!

5. **Don't waste the pulp.** One of the downsides of juicing is that it removes a significant amount of fiber from produce in the form of pulp. You can reap the nutritional benefits of this pulp by stirring a small amount of it into your finished juice. You can even use it in place of fats like butter or oil in recipes for your favorite baked goods!

6. **Drink it down quickly.** This doesn't mean that you should chug your juice straight from the juicer—it simply means that the longer you wait to drink your fresh juice, the more nutritional value will be lost. Try to make only as much juice as you can drink in one sitting, and definitely don't store it for more than two or three days. Also, always use ripe fruit and vegetables to get the most nutrients from your food.

7. **Store your juice correctly.** If you do have to store extra juice, make sure you do it right. Don't just place a glass of juice in the refrigerator to keep, as this will result in oxidation and loss of vital nutrients. Rather, store fresh juice in an airtight container (ideally glass rather than plastic). Filling the container all the way to the top will also help to prevent nutrient loss.

8. **Don't be afraid to get creative.** One of the main reasons people fall off the wagon with diets is that they get bored. If you prepare the same juice each and every day, it will eventually lose its novelty (and you'll also be depriving yourself of vital nutrients). Don't be afraid to use new ingredients that you've never tried before. They may not always work out, but you will likely discover some delicious flavor combinations along the way!

9. **Take advantage of seasonal produce.** Keep an eye out for sales at your local grocery store, and don't be a stranger at farmers' markets in your area. Summer and fall are the ideal times to take advantage of fresh, local produce. You can also save a lot of money by buying directly from the farm or farmer over grocery store prices. Many farms

offer a community-shared agriculture (CSA) program, through which they'll deliver a box of fresh produce straight to your door every week.

10. **Have fun with it.** If you think of juicing as a necessary evil or simply as a means to lose weight, you may find it a difficult habit to stick to. You'd do better to think of juicing as a fun and easy way to increase your daily fruit and vegetable intake. Think about all of the amazing benefits your body will gain from drinking fresh-pressed juices!

PART FOUR

175 Healthful Juicing Recipes

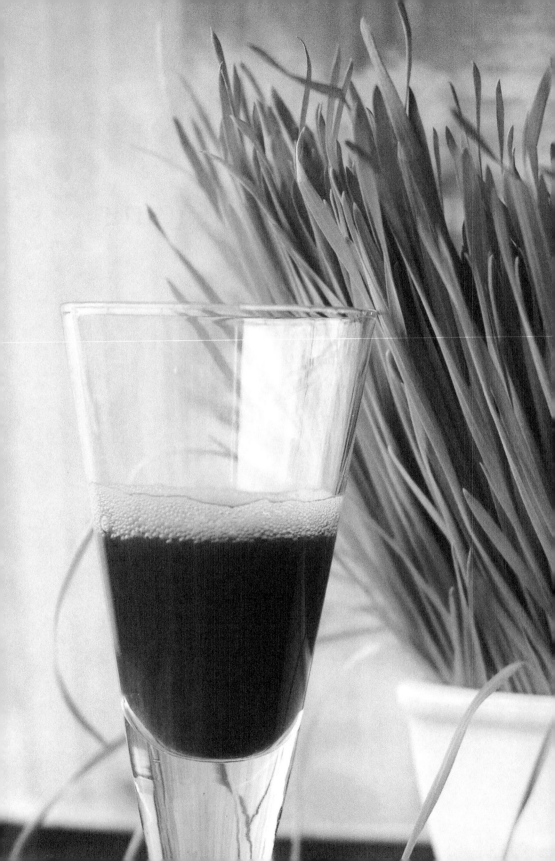

CHAPTER THIRTEEN

40 Green Juices

Rousing Raspberry Radish Juice

This recipe is packed with energy-boosting ingredients that will help to power you through your day.

6 MEDIUM RADISHES, GREENS INCLUDED
2 MEDIUM PEARS
1 CUP RASPBERRIES
1 CUP BROCCOLI FLORETS
1 SMALL BUNCH FRESH MUSTARD GREENS

1. Trim or chop the ingredients as needed to fit into the feed chute of your juicer.

2. Place a pitcher or container under the spout of the juicer.

3. Feed the ingredients through the juicer in the order listed.

4. Stir the juice briefly; then pour it into glasses and serve immediately.

5. Fresh juice may be refrigerated in an airtight container for up to 3 days.

Summer Celery Cucumber Juice

Cucumbers have a very high water content that makes them ideal for juicing. Additionally, cucumbers are known for containing potassium and phytosterol, both of which make them beneficial for reducing bad cholesterol.

2 HOTHOUSE CUCUMBERS
4 LARGE STALKS CELERY, GREENS INCLUDED
1 SMALL HEAD BROCCOLI
1 LARGE GRANNY SMITH APPLE

1. Trim or chop the ingredients as needed to fit into the feed chute of your juicer.

2. Place a pitcher or container under the spout of the juicer.

3. Feed the ingredients through the juicer in the order listed.

4. Stir the juice briefly; then pour it into glasses and serve immediately.

5. Fresh juice may be refrigerated in an airtight container for up to 3 days.

Purple Cabbage Grapefruit Juice

The combination of purple cabbage and grapefruit gives this recipe a unique color, not to mention delicious flavor.

2 LARGE LEAVES ROMAINE LETTUCE
1 SMALL HEAD PURPLE CABBAGE
1 MEDIUM PINK GRAPEFRUIT, HALVED AND PEELED
1 CUP CHERRIES, PITTED

1. Trim or chop the ingredients as needed to fit into the feed chute of your juicer.

2. Place a pitcher or container under the spout of the juicer.

3. Feed the ingredients through the juicer in the order listed.

4. Stir the juice briefly; then pour it into glasses and serve immediately.

5. Fresh juice may be refrigerated in an airtight container for up to 3 days.

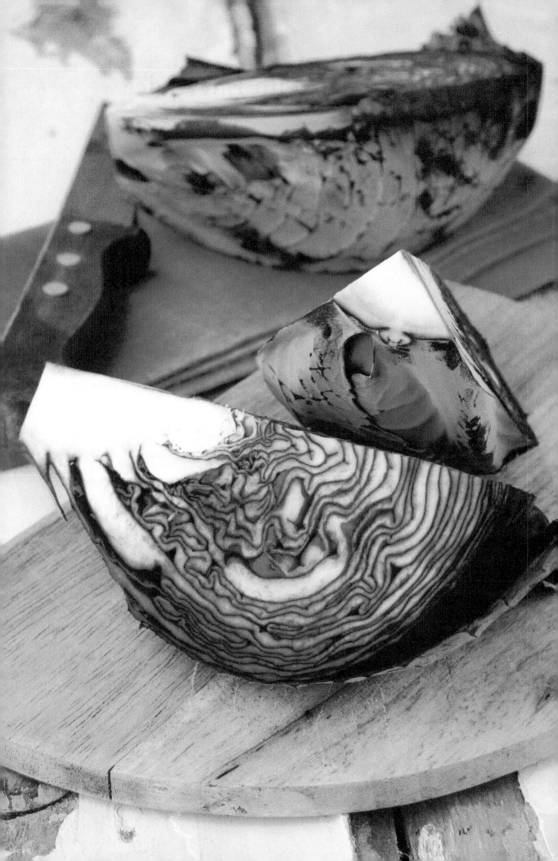

Green with Envy Juice

This juice blend is a delightful mixture of healthful greens. The parsley enhances the flavor and boosts the vitamin C content. Parsley also contains folate, which helps improve heart health and prevent certain cancers.

1 BUNCH OR 2 CUPS SPINACH LEAVES
1 HOTHOUSE CUCUMBER
1 GREEN BELL PEPPER
1 LARGE LEAF CURLY KALE
½ BUNCH FRESH CURLY PARSLEY

1. Trim or chop the ingredients as needed to fit into the feed chute of your juicer.

2. Place a pitcher or container under the spout of the juicer.

3. Feed the ingredients through the juicer in the order listed.

4. Stir the juice briefly; then pour it into glasses and serve immediately.

5. Fresh juice may be refrigerated in an airtight container for up to 3 days.

Lemon Lime Green Juice

MAKES 3 SERVINGS, 8 TO 10 OUNCES EACH

Don't let the dark green color of this juice fool you—it's full of light, citrusy flavor.

3 LARGE LEMONS, HALVED AND PEELED

2 SMALL LIMES, HALVED AND PEELED

1 BUNCH FRESH PARSLEY

1 MEDIUM PEAR

1 MEDIUM APPLE

½ BUNCH FRESH CILANTRO

1. Trim or chop the ingredients as needed to fit into the feed chute of your juicer.

2. Place a pitcher or container under the spout of the juicer.

3. Feed the ingredients through the juicer in the order listed.

4. Stir the juice briefly; then pour it into glasses and serve immediately.

5. Fresh juice may be refrigerated in an airtight container for up to 3 days.

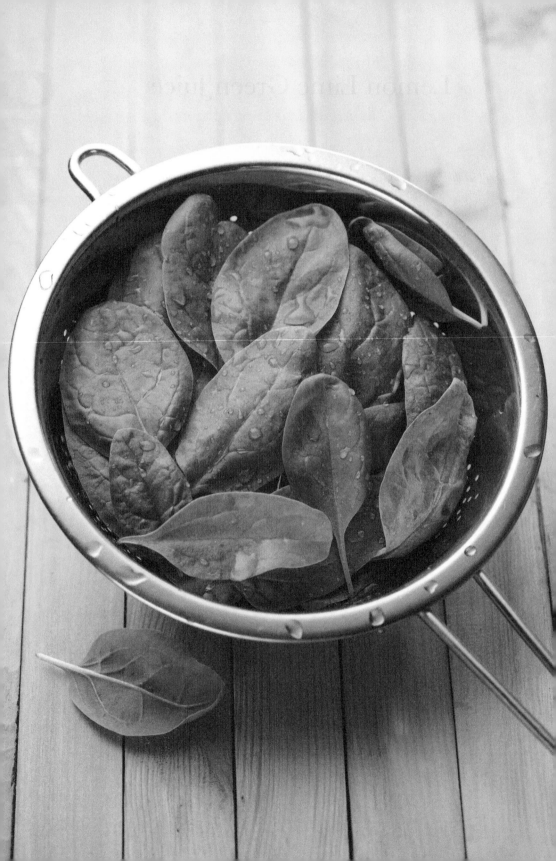

Spinach Basil Lime Juice

MAKES 3 SERVINGS, 8 TO 10 OUNCES EACH

In this recipe, the flavors of basil and lime combine perfectly with fresh spinach to make a refreshing and nutritious beverage.

....

1 BUNCH OR 2 CUPS SPINACH LEAVES
½ BUNCH FRESH BASIL LEAVES
1 SMALL LIME, HALVED AND PEELED

....

1. Place a pitcher or container under the spout of the feed chute of your juicer.

2. Feed the ingredients through the juicer in the order listed.

3. Stir the juice briefly; then pour it into glasses and serve immediately.

4. Fresh juice may be refrigerated in an airtight container for up to 3 days.

Tropical Sunrise Green Juice

This delightful green juice provides you with all the benefits of leafy greens, but all you'll taste is the flavor of tropical paradise.

2 KIWIS, PEELED
2 LARGE LEAVES CURLY KALE
1 BUNCH OR 2 CUPS COLLARD GREENS
1 MANGO, PITTED
½ SMALL PINEAPPLE, CORED AND HUSKED

1. Trim or chop the ingredients as needed to fit into the feed chute of your juicer.

2. Place a pitcher or container under the spout of the juicer.

3. Feed the ingredients through the juicer in the order listed.

4. Stir the juice briefly; then pour it into glasses and serve immediately.

5. Fresh juice may be refrigerated in an airtight container for up to 3 days.

True Blue Vegetable Tonic

MAKES 3 SERVINGS, 8 TO 10 OUNCES EACH

This recipe gets its name from several elements. Not only do the blueberries give this recipe a blue color, but the addition of spirulina (blue-green algae) ups the nutrient content.

1 CUP BROCCOLI FLORETS
1 CUP CAULIFLOWER FLORETS
1 CUP BLUEBERRIES
1 SMALL BULB FENNEL, GREENS INCLUDED
1 MEDIUM APPLE
1 TABLESPOON SPIRULINA POWDER

1. Trim or chop the ingredients as needed to fit into the feed chute of your juicer.

2. Place a pitcher or container under the spout of the juicer.

3. Feed the first 5 ingredients through the juicer in the order listed.

4. Stir the spirulina powder into the juice, then pour the juice into glasses and serve immediately.

5. Fresh juice may be refrigerated in an airtight container for up to 3 days.

Blueberry Banana Booster

Banana can be a tricky fruit to juice because it is so much softer than many fruits. For this reason, it's important that you juice the ingredients in the order listed—the more structured vegetables will help push the soft banana through the juicer.

1 PINT FRESH BLUEBERRIES
1 MEDIUM BANANA, PEELED
1 LARGE CARROT
½ SEEDLESS CUCUMBER

1. Trim or chop the ingredients as needed to fit into the feed chute of your juicer.

2. Place a pitcher or container under the spout of the juicer.

3. Feed the ingredients through the juicer in the order listed.

4. Stir the juice briefly; then pour it into glasses and serve immediately.

5. Fresh juice may be refrigerated in an airtight container for up to 3 days.

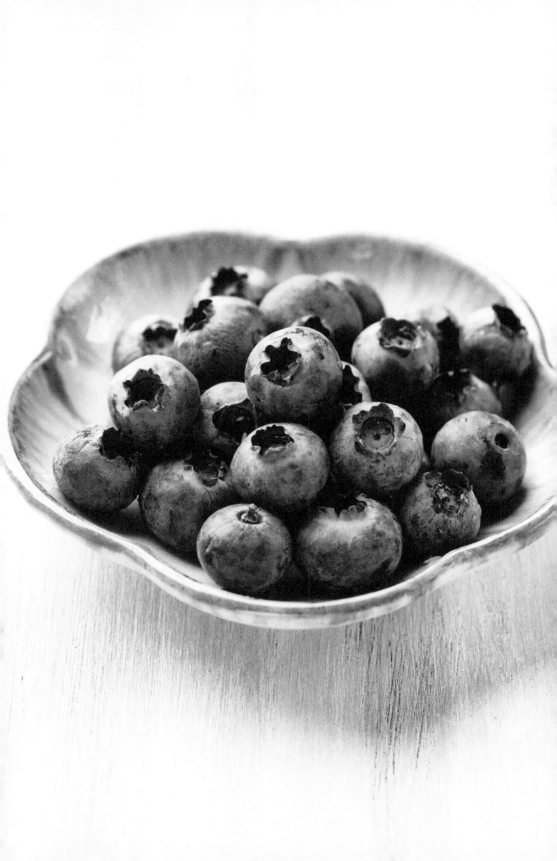

Kiwi Apple Cucumber Juice

Cucumbers are a popular juice ingredient due to their high water content. In this recipe they provide the perfect backdrop to support the flavors of kiwi and apple.

1 LARGE ENGLISH CUCUMBER
2 MEDIUM APPLES
2 KIWIS, PEELED

1. Trim or chop the ingredients as needed to fit into the feed chute of your juicer.

2. Place a pitcher or container under the spout of the juicer.

3. Feed the ingredients through the juicer in the order listed.

4. Stir the juice briefly; then pour it into glasses and serve immediately.

5. Fresh juice may be refrigerated in an airtight container for up to 3 days.

Good Morning Grape Celery Juice

Grapes are known for their crispness and tart flavor. In this recipe, they provide these benefits and more! Grapes are also known for their antioxidant and anti-inflammatory benefits.

4 LARGE STALKS CELERY
2 CUPS SEEDLESS GREEN GRAPES
1 SMALL SCALLION
1 SMALL APPLE

1. Trim or chop the ingredients as needed to fit into the feed chute of your juicer.

2. Place a pitcher or container under the spout of the juicer.

3. Feed the ingredients through the juicer in the order listed.

4. Stir the juice briefly; then pour it into glasses and serve immediately.

5. Fresh juice may be refrigerated in an airtight container for up to 3 days.

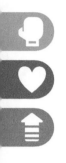

Seriously Green Juice Blend

Don't let the name of this juice frighten you—the only thing serious about it is the health benefits it offers.

2 LARGE STALKS CELERY
2 NAVEL ORANGES, HALVED AND PEELED
1 SMALL ENGLISH CUCUMBER
½ BUNCH OR 2 CUPS COLLARD GREENS
½ BUNCH OR 2 CUPS SPINACH LEAVES
½ SMALL LIME, PEELED

1. Trim or chop the ingredients as needed to fit into the feed chute of your juicer.

2. Place a pitcher or container under the spout of the juicer.

3. Feed the ingredients through the juicer in the order listed.

4. Stir the juice briefly; then pour it into glasses and serve immediately.

5. Fresh juice may be refrigerated in an airtight container for up to 3 days.

Blood Orange Swiss Chard Juice

Swiss chard sometimes has a bitter taste to it, which is why blood oranges are so essential in this recipe—they boost the nutrient content while also disguising the flavor of the Swiss chard.

2 MEDIUM BLOOD ORANGES, HALVED AND PEELED
2 STALKS CELERY
1 MEDIUM CARROT
1 BUNCH OR 2 CUPS SWISS CHARD

1. Trim or chop the ingredients as needed to fit into the feed chute of your juicer.

2. Place a pitcher or container under the spout of the juicer.

3. Feed the ingredients through the juicer in the order listed.

4. Stir the juice briefly; then pour it into glasses and serve immediately.

5. Fresh juice may be refrigerated in an airtight container for up to 3 days.

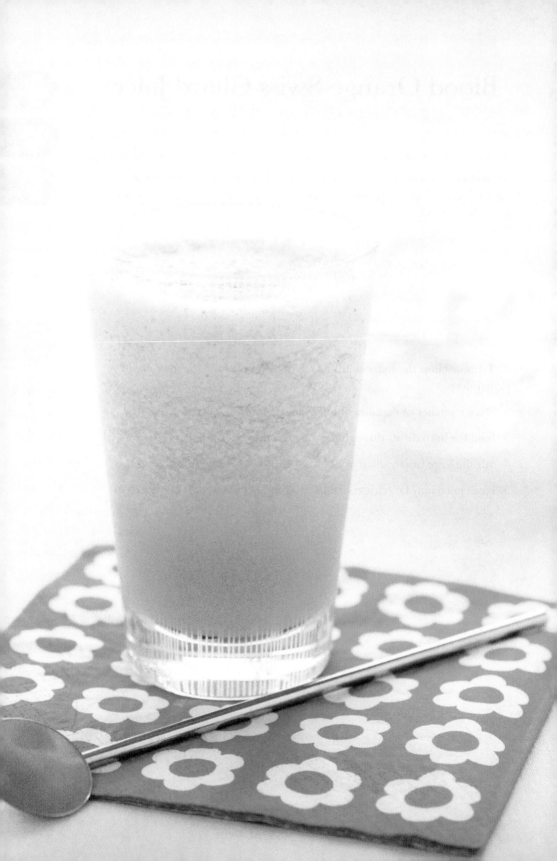

Pineapple Celery Juice

Both celery and pineapple are known for their detoxifying qualities. In this recipe, the subtle flavor of celery provides the perfect backdrop for the sweetness of pineapple and a hint of freshness from the cilantro.

6 LARGE STALKS CELERY
½ PINEAPPLE, CORED AND HUSKED
2 TO 3 SPRIGS FRESH CILANTRO

1. Trim or chop the ingredients as needed to fit into the feed chute of your juicer.

2. Place a pitcher or container under the spout of the juicer.

3. Feed the ingredients through the juicer in the order listed.

4. Stir the juice briefly; then pour it into glasses and serve immediately.

5. Fresh juice may be refrigerated in an airtight container for up to 3 days.

Berry Brussels Sprouts Juice Blend

MAKES 3 TO 4 SERVINGS, 8 TO 10 OUNCES EACH

Brussels sprouts don't have a lot of fans, but they're a valuable source of dietary fiber, folate, and manganese. In this recipe you get all the benefits of Brussels sprouts with the flavor of berries.

2 LARGE LEAVES ROMAINE LETTUCE
8 BRUSSELS SPROUTS, TRIMMED
1 CUP STRAWBERRIES
1 CUP BLACKBERRIES
½ LIME, PEELED

1. Trim or chop the ingredients as needed to fit into the feed chute of your juicer.

2. Place a pitcher or container under the spout of the juicer.

3. Feed the ingredients through the juicer in the order listed.

4. Stir the juice briefly; then pour it into glasses and serve immediately.

5. Fresh juice may be refrigerated in an airtight container for up to 3 days.

Cilantro Spinach Lime Juice

This juice is incredibly refreshing, not to mention full of nutrients. In addition to its fresh flavor, cilantro is also known for its antioxidant content, which helps lower bad cholesterol and raise good cholesterol.

2 BUNCHES OR 4 CUPS SPINACH
½ BUNCH FRESH CILANTRO
1 LIME, HALVED AND PEELED

1. Trim or chop the ingredients as needed to fit into the feed chute of your juicer.

2. Place a pitcher or container under the spout of the juicer.

3. Feed the ingredients through the juicer in the order listed.

4. Stir the juice briefly; then pour it into glasses and serve immediately.

5. Fresh juice may be refrigerated in an airtight container for up to 3 days.

Grapefruit Ginger Green Juice

Grapefruit offers a tangy yet sweet flavor in addition to a number of vital nutrients. Pink grapefruit in particular contains phytonutrients like lycopene (also found in tomatoes), an antioxidant that has been shown to reduce tumor growth.

3 MEDIUM PINK GRAPEFRUIT, HALVED AND PEELED
2 LARGE LEAVES ROMAINE LETTUCE
1 LARGE STALK CELERY
1 INCH GINGERROOT

1. Trim or chop the ingredients as needed to fit into the feed chute of your juicer.

2. Place a pitcher or container under the spout of the juicer.

3. Feed the ingredients through the juicer in the order listed.

4. Stir the juice briefly; then pour it into glasses and serve immediately.

5. Fresh juice may be refrigerated in an airtight container for up to 3 days.

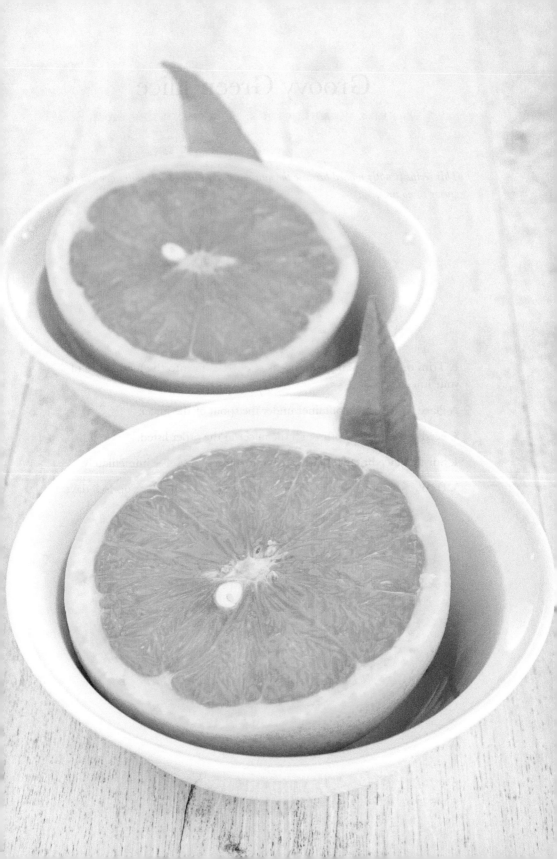

Groovy Green Juice

This recipe is aptly named because the nutrient-packed ingredients will have you feeling groovy in no time.

2 NAVEL ORANGES, HALVED AND PEELED
1 CUP RED SEEDLESS GRAPES
2 MEDIUM SCALLIONS
1 SMALL HEAD BOK CHOY
½ SMALL HEAD GREEN CABBAGE

1. Trim or chop the ingredients as needed to fit into the feed chute of your juicer.

2. Place a pitcher or container under the spout of the juicer.

3. Feed the ingredients through the juicer in the order listed.

4. Stir the juice briefly; then pour it into glasses and serve immediately.

5. Fresh juice may be refrigerated in an airtight container for up to 3 days.

Sweet and Simple Juice Blend

This juice recipe is exactly what it sounds like: sweet and simple. Just combine a few handfuls each of collard greens and cabbage with a fresh orange and apple to create this lightly sweetened juice blend.

1 BUNCH OR 2 CUPS COLLARD GREENS
1 SMALL HEAD GREEN CABBAGE
1 MEDIUM APPLE
1 MEDIUM NAVEL ORANGE, HALVED AND PEELED

1. Trim or chop the ingredients as needed to fit into the feed chute of your juicer.

2. Place a pitcher or container under the spout of the juicer.

3. Feed the ingredients through the juicer in the order listed.

4. Stir the juice briefly; then pour it into glasses and serve immediately.

5. Fresh juice may be refrigerated in an airtight container for up to 3 days.

115

40 GREEN JUICES

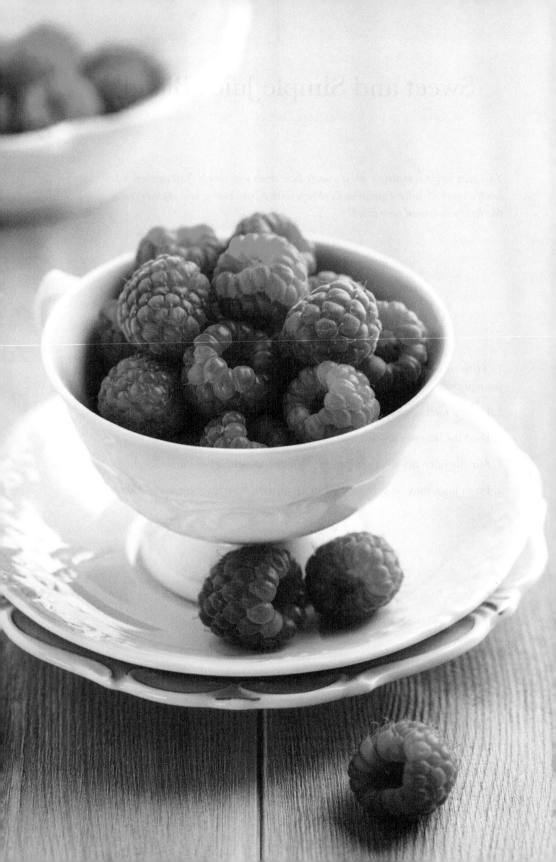

Raspberry Spinach Refresher

Everything about this recipe screams "refreshing," from the crisp flavor of spinach to the sweetness of raspberries and the coolness of cilantro.

2 CUPS RASPBERRIES
1 BUNCH OR 2 CUPS SPINACH LEAVES
1 SMALL LIME, HALVED AND PEELED
2 TO 3 SPRIGS FRESH CILANTRO

1. Trim or chop the ingredients as needed to fit into the feed chute of your juicer.

2. Place a pitcher or container under the spout of the juicer.

3. Feed the ingredients through the juicer in the order listed.

4. Stir the juice briefly; then pour it into glasses and serve immediately.

5. Fresh juice may be refrigerated in an airtight container for up to 3 days.

Triple Berry Tonic

This recipe includes the trifecta of fresh berries: blueberries, strawberries, and raspberries. If that isn't enough, try adding a splash of sparkling water.

2 CUPS BLUEBERRIES
2 LARGE ROMAINE LETTUCE LEAVES
1 CUP STRAWBERRIES
1 CUP RASPBERRIES
1 LARGE STALK CELERY
SPLASH OF SPARKLING WATER (OPTIONAL)

1. Trim or chop the ingredients as needed to fit into the feed chute of your juicer.

2. Place a pitcher or container under the spout of the juicer.

3. Feed the first 5 ingredients through the juicer in the order listed.

4. Stir the juice briefly; then pour it into glasses and serve immediately, with a splash of sparkling water (if using).

5. Fresh juice may be refrigerated in an airtight container for up to 3 days.

Pick-Me-Up Green Juice Blend

This recipe is full of ingredients that will pick you up and give you the energy you need to get through the rest of your day.

2 KIWIS, PEELED
1 BUNCH OR 2 CUPS DANDELION GREENS
1 SMALL KOHLRABI
1 HANDFUL SUGAR SNAP PEAS
1 MEDIUM APPLE

1. Trim or chop the ingredients as needed to fit into the feed chute of your juicer.

2. Place a pitcher or container under the spout of the juicer.

3. Feed the ingredients through the juicer in the order listed.

4. Stir the juice briefly; then pour it into glasses and serve immediately.

5. Fresh juice may be refrigerated in an airtight container for up to 3 days.

Wonderful Watermelon Wake-Up

Made with sweet watermelon and fresh orange juice, this recipe is just what you need to wake up in the morning. Enjoy it on a regular day or serve it up special for a Sunday brunch.

1 SMALL SEEDLESS WATERMELON, RIND REMOVED
2 NAVEL ORANGES, QUARTERED
HANDFUL OF MINT LEAVES
ICE TO SERVE

1. Chop the watermelon as needed to fit into the feed chute of your juicer.

2. Place a pitcher or container under the spout of the juicer.

3. Feed the watermelon through the juicer.

4. Squeeze two orange quarters into each of 4 glasses, dropping the peels into the glass.

5. Add a few mint leaves to each glass and fill with ice.

6. Pour the watermelon juice evenly into the 4 glasses and serve immediately.

7. Fresh juice may be refrigerated in an airtight container for up to 3 days.

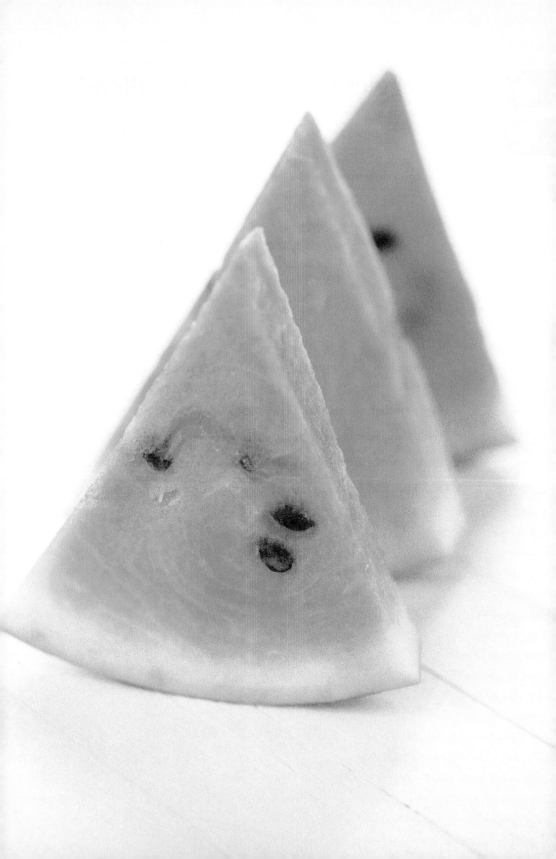

Veggies and More Juice Blend

This recipe is exactly what it sounds like: a wealth of delicious vegetables and much more.

1 CUP CAULIFLOWER FLORETS

1 MEDIUM TURNIP

1 SMALL PARSNIP

½ BUNCH OR 2 CUPS SWISS CHARD

½ BUNCH FRESH PARSLEY

½ SMALL PINEAPPLE, CORED AND HUSKED

1. Trim or chop the ingredients as needed to fit into the feed chute of your juicer.

2. Place a pitcher or container under the spout of the juicer.

3. Feed the ingredients through the juicer in the order listed.

4. Stir the juice briefly; then pour it into glasses and serve immediately.

5. Fresh juice may be refrigerated in an airtight container for up to 3 days.

Take Charge Turnip Booster

Turnips are a root vegetable known for their high concentration of calcium, magnesium, and potassium. They've also been shown to have anti-cancer benefits.

2 MEDIUM TURNIPS, GREENS INCLUDED
2 LARGE STALKS CELERY
1 LARGE CARROT
1 MEDIUM APPLE
1 MEDIUM NAVEL ORANGE, HALVED AND PEELED
½ LIME, PEELED

1. Trim or chop the ingredients as needed to fit into the feed chute of your juicer.

2. Place a pitcher or container under the spout of the juicer.

3. Feed the ingredients through the juicer in the order listed.

4. Stir the juice briefly; then pour it into glasses and serve immediately.

5. Fresh juice may be refrigerated in an airtight container for up to 3 days.

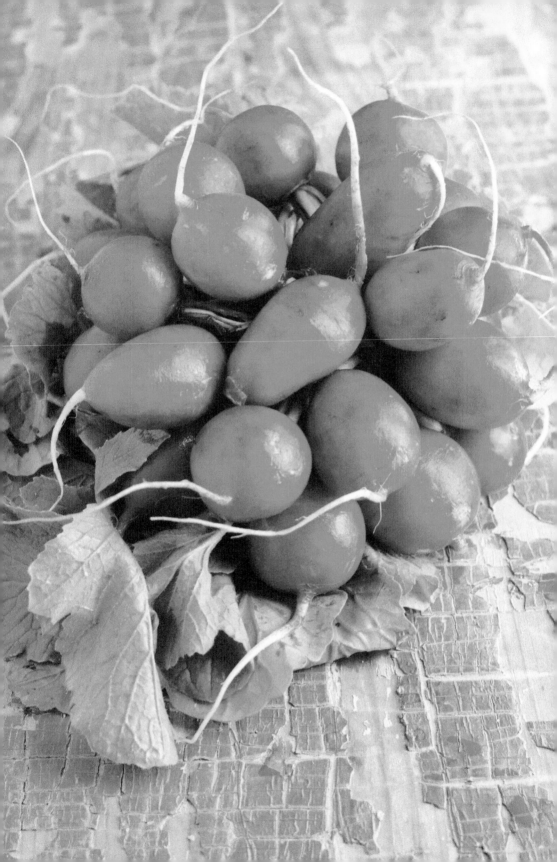

Red and Green Radish Juice

When you think of vegetables for juicing, radishes may not be the first thing that comes to mind. Radishes are, however, a wonderful option for juicing because they're full of flavor not to mention protein, folic acid, vitamin C, and other vital nutrients.

10 SMALL RADISHES, GREENS INCLUDED
2 CUPS CHOPPED KALE LEAVES
2 LARGE STALKS CELERY, GREENS INCLUDED
1 LARGE CARROT
1 NAVEL ORANGE, HALVED AND PEELED

1. Trim or chop the ingredients as needed to fit into the feed chute of your juicer.

2. Place a pitcher or container under the spout of the juicer.

3. Feed the ingredients through the juicer in the order listed.

4. Stir the juice briefly; then pour it into glasses and serve immediately.

5. Fresh juice may be refrigerated in an airtight container for up to 3 days.

Cilantro Coconut Chiller

This chiller is quick and easy to prepare. It's a wonderful option if you are looking for something cool and refreshing to enjoy on a hot summer day by the pool.

1 BUNCH FRESH CILANTRO
1 LIME, HALVED AND PEELED
4 CUPS CHILLED COCONUT WATER

1. Place a pitcher or container under the spout of the juicer.

2. Feed the cilantro through the juicer, then the lime.

3. Stir the coconut water into the juice, then pour the juice into glasses and serve immediately.

4. Fresh juice may be refrigerated in an airtight container for up to 3 days.

Jazzy Juice Blend

Dandelion greens, like most leafy greens, are an excellent source of iron and calcium. What makes this recipe unique, however, is the flavor of starfruit.

1 BUNCH OR 2 CUPS DANDELION GREENS
2 SMALL TURNIPS, GREENS INCLUDED
1 CUP CAULIFLOWER
2 MEDIUM STARFRUIT
1 MEDIUM APPLE

1. Trim or chop the ingredients as needed to fit into the feed chute of your juicer.

2. Place a pitcher or container under the spout of the juicer.

3. Feed the ingredients through the juicer in the order listed.

4. Stir the juice briefly; then pour it into glasses and serve immediately.

5. Fresh juice may be refrigerated in an airtight container for up to 3 days.

Cucumber Apple Kale Juice

Cucumber is known for its high water content and detoxifying qualities. Apples, on the other hand, are known for their high concentration of phytonutrients, which help to regulate blood sugar levels—a benefit particularly valuable for diabetics.

1 LARGE ENGLISH CUCUMBER
2 MEDIUM GOLDEN DELICIOUS APPLES
2 LARGE LEAVES CURLY KALE

1. Trim or chop the ingredients as needed to fit into the feed chute of your juicer.

2. Place a pitcher or container under the spout of the juicer.

3. Feed the ingredients through the juicer in the order listed.

4. Stir the juice briefly; then pour it into glasses and serve immediately.

5. Fresh juice may be refrigerated in an airtight container for up to 3 days.

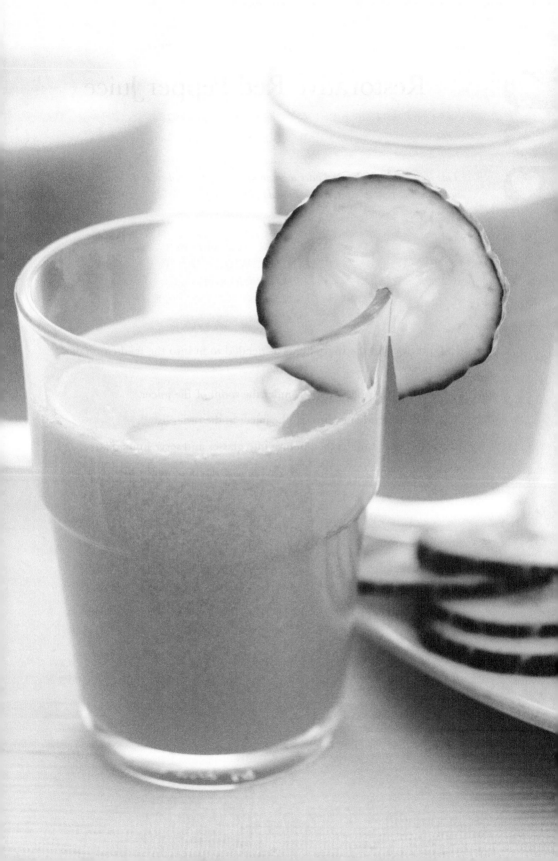

Restorative Red Pepper Juice

This recipe yields a flavorful juice with an appealing dark red color. If you feel like you need to sweeten it up a bit, feel free to add another apple.

2 MEDIUM RED BELL PEPPERS
1 CUP CHOPPED RED CABBAGE
1 LARGE CARROT
1 MEDIUM GRANNY SMITH APPLE

1. Trim or chop the ingredients as needed to fit into the feed chute of your juicer.

2. Place a pitcher or container under the spout of the juicer.

3. Feed the ingredients through the juicer in the order listed.

4. Stir the juice briefly; then pour it into glasses and serve immediately.

5. Fresh juice may be refrigerated in an airtight container for up to 3 days.

Clean Celery Carrot Juice

Both carrots and celery are known for their detoxifying qualities. Combined with other detoxifying ingredients like cauliflower and blueberries, this makes one powerful recipe.

4 LARGE STALKS CELERY
2 LARGE CARROTS
1 CUP CAULIFLOWER FLORETS
1 CUP BLUEBERRIES
1 BLOOD ORANGE, HALVED AND PEELED

1. Trim or chop the ingredients as needed to fit into the feed chute of your juicer.

2. Place a pitcher or container under the spout of the juicer.

3. Feed the ingredients through the juicer in the order listed.

4. Stir the juice briefly; then pour it into glasses and serve immediately.

5. Fresh juice may be refrigerated in an airtight container for up to 3 days.

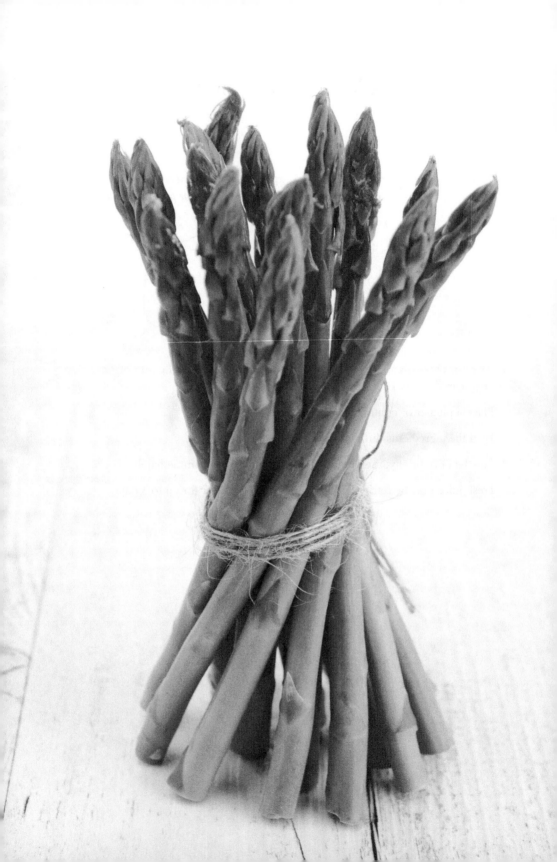

Get Your Juices Flowing

Asparagus and snap peas are both energy-boosting vegetables while kiwi and pineapple help cleanse and detoxify your body. The combination will keep you going strong throughout the day.

2 KIWIS, PEELED
1 BUNCH OR 20 ASPARAGUS SPEARS, ENDS TRIMMED
1 HANDFUL SUGAR SNAP PEAS
½ SMALL PINEAPPLE, CORED AND HUSKED

1. Trim or chop the ingredients as needed to fit into the feed chute of your juicer.

2. Place a pitcher or container under the spout of the juicer.

3. Feed the ingredients through the juicer in the order listed.

4. Stir the juice briefly; then pour it into glasses and serve immediately.

5. Fresh juice may be refrigerated in an airtight container for up to 3 days.

Lovely Lemon Lavender Infusion

The tartness of lemon and the calming benefits of lavender may seem to be at odds with each other, but they blend well in this unique recipe.

1 BUNCH OR 2 CUPS BABY SPINACH
2 MEDIUM LEMONS, HALVED AND PEELED
1 CUP BLACKBERRIES
2 TEASPOONS DRIED LAVENDER

1. Trim or chop the ingredients as needed to fit into the feed chute of your juicer.

2. Place a pitcher or container under the spout of the juicer.

3. Feed the first 3 ingredients through the juicer in the order listed.

4. Stir the dried lavender into the juice, then pour the juice into glasses and serve immediately.

5. Fresh juice may be refrigerated in an airtight container for up to 3 days.

Marvelous Mango Green Juice

This recipe provides you with all the health benefits associated with kale and romaine lettuce while you get to enjoy the flavor of ripe mango.

2 MANGOS, PITTED
2 LARGE LEAVES KALE
1 BUNCH OR 2 CUPS ROMAINE LETTUCE
1 SCALLION

1. Trim or chop the ingredients as needed to fit into the feed chute of your juicer.

2. Place a pitcher or container under the spout of the juicer.

3. Feed the ingredients through the juicer in the order listed.

4. Stir the juice briefly; then pour it into glasses and serve immediately.

5. Fresh juice may be refrigerated in an airtight container for up to 3 days.

Garden Greens Juice Blend

MAKES 2 TO 3 SERVINGS, 8 TO 10 OUNCES EACH

This recipe is the perfect opportunity to use the fresh greens from your backyard herb garden. If you don't have your own garden, visit your local farmers' market or health food store for the freshest produce.

1 BUNCH OR 2 CUPS SPRING GREENS
2 LARGE LEAVES CURLY KALE
2 LARGE LEAVES ROMAINE LETTUCE
2 TO 3 SPRIGS FRESH MINT
2 TO 3 SPRIGS FRESH PARSLEY
2 TO 3 SPRIGS FRESH CILANTRO

1. Trim or chop the ingredients as needed to fit into the feed chute of your juicer.

2. Place a pitcher or container under the spout of the juicer.

3. Feed the ingredients through the juicer in the order listed.

4. Stir the juice briefly; then pour it into glasses and serve immediately.

5. Fresh juice may be refrigerated in an airtight container for up to 3 days.

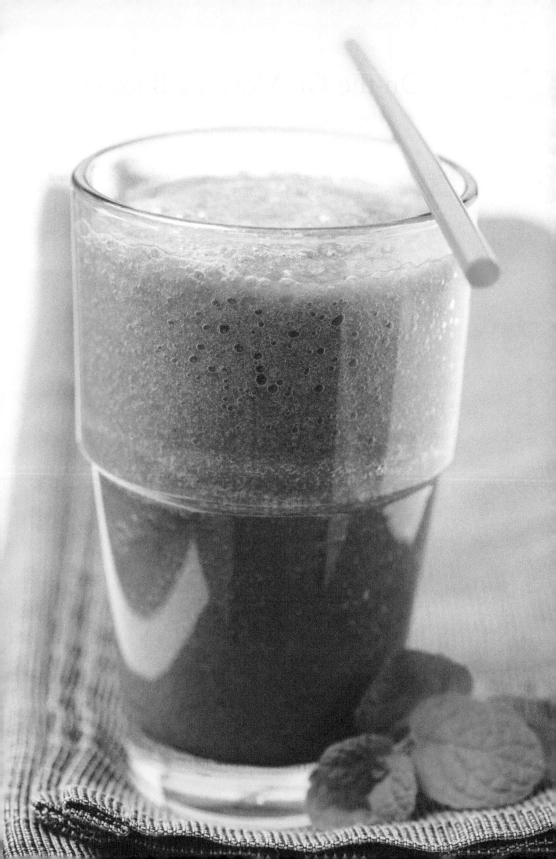

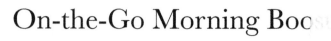

On-the-Go Morning Boost

The ingredients in this recipe are known for their energy-boosting qualities
something to get you going in the morning, reach for a glass of this green

1 BUNCH OR 2 CUPS COLLARD GREENS
2 SMALL KOHLRABI, GREENS INCLUDED
1 CUP BROCCOLI FLORETS
1 MEDIUM APPLE
1 MEDIUM PEAR

1. Trim or chop the ingredients as needed to fit into the feed chute of your juicer.

2. Place a pitcher or container under the spout of the juicer.

3. Feed the ingredients through the juicer in the order listed.

4. Stir the juice briefly; then pour it into glasses and serve immediately.

5. Fresh juice may be refrigerated in an airtight container for up to 3 days.

Refreshing Romaine
and Radish Juice

Unlike other lettuces such as iceberg, romaine is packed with nutrients. It's rich in vitamins A, C, and K as well as minerals, including iron, potassium, manganese, and magnesium.

1 HEAD ROMAINE LETTUCE
6 SMALL RADISHES, GREENS INCLUDED
1 LARGE LEAF RED CHARD
1 MEDIUM APPLE
4 TO 5 SPRIGS FRESH CILANTRO

1. Trim or chop the ingredients as needed to fit into the feed chute of your juicer.

2. Place a pitcher or container under the spout of the juicer.

3. Feed the ingredients through the juicer in the order listed.

4. Stir the juice briefly; then pour it into glasses and serve immediately.

5. Fresh juice may be refrigerated in an airtight container for up to 3 days.

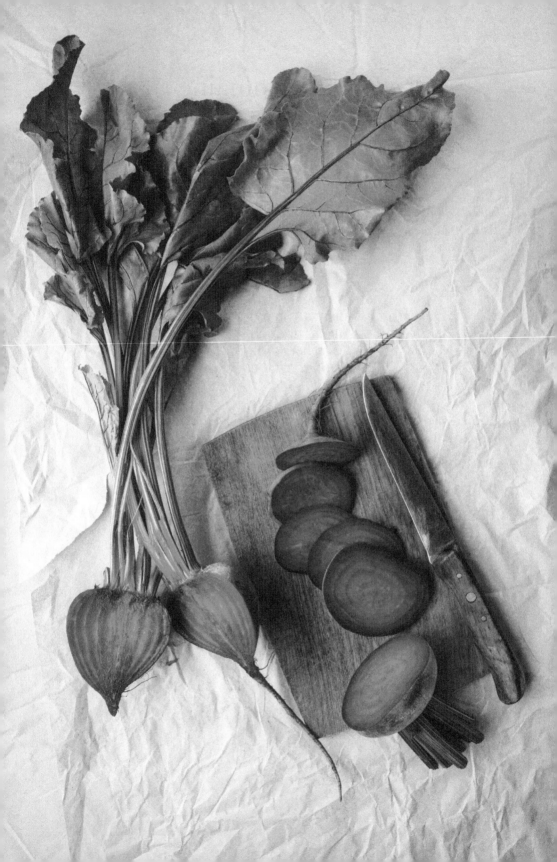

Broccoli Beet Blast

Beets have been shown to help oxygenate the blood, which is essential to improving exercise performance and recovery. Beets also contain iron, choline, manganese, and a number of vitamins. These nutrients are more concentrated in the greens, so don't forget to include them in your juice as well!

1 SMALL HEAD BROCCOLI, CUT INTO SPEARS
2 MEDIUM BEETS, GREENS INCLUDED
1 CUP RASPBERRIES OR BLUEBERRIES
5 TO 6 FRESH BASIL LEAVES

1. Trim or chop the ingredients as needed to fit into the feed chute of your juicer.

2. Place a pitcher or plastic container under the spout of the juicer.

3. Feed the ingredients through the juicer in the order listed.

4. Stir the juice briefly; then pour it into glasses and serve immediately.

5. Fresh juice may be refrigerated in an airtight container for up to 3 days.

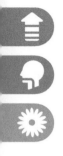

Arugula Ginger Green Juice

MAKES 2 TO 3 SERVINGS, 8 TO 10 OUNCES EACH

Arugula is a type of lettuce rich in both antioxidants and flavonoids. It also contains a variety of essential vitamins and minerals to support healthful bodily function.

1 BUNCH OR 2 CUPS ARUGULA
2 LARGE RED KALE LEAVES
1 SMALL CUCUMBER
1 LARGE STALK CELERY, GREENS INCLUDED
1 INCH GINGERROOT

1. Trim or chop the ingredients as needed to fit into the feed chute of your juicer.

2. Place a pitcher or container under the spout of the juicer.

3. Feed the ingredients through the juicer in the order listed.

4. Stir the juice briefly; then pour it into glasses and serve immediately.

5. Fresh juice may be refrigerated in an airtight container for up to 3 days.

Get Your Greens Here

Leafy greens, like those included in this recipe, are known for being powerhouses of nutrition. They're an excellent source of iron, vitamin K, and calcium as well as other vitamins and minerals.

2 LARGE LEAVES KALE
2 LARGE LEAVES ROMAINE LETTUCE
1 SMALL BUNCH OR 2 CUPS SPINACH
½ BUNCH OR 1 CUP DANDELION GREENS

1. Trim or chop the ingredients as needed to fit into the feed chute of your juicer.

2. Place a pitcher or container under the spout of the juicer.

3. Feed the ingredients through the juicer in the order listed.

4. Stir the juice briefly; then pour it into glasses and serve immediately.

5. Fresh juice may be refrigerated in an airtight container for up to 3 days.

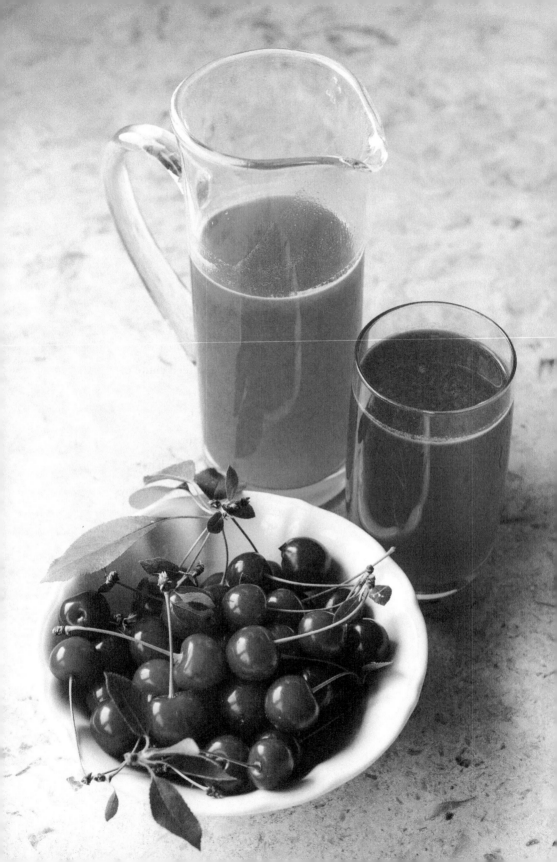

CHAPTER **FOURTEEN**

45 Fruit Juices

Orange Blossom Juice

Pineapple Apple Juice

Cran-Raspberry Spritzer

Sweet and Shocking Juice

Strawberry Watermelon Juice

Honeyed Cantaloupe Tonic

Sparkling Citrus Juice

Pretty in Pink

Black Cherry Basil Blast

Morning Melon Wake-Up Juice

Peachy Pomegranate Juice

Cucumber Melon Cooler

Cherry Berry Blast

Calming Tropical Juice Blend

Soothing Strawberry Juice

Gooseberry Goodness

Fruity Fennel Juice Blend

Kiwi Lime Spritzer

Minty Melon Juice Blend

Merry Mango Juice

Lemongrass Apple Juice

Orange Lavender Juice

Passion Fruit Crush

Very Berry Juice Blend

Royal-Red Raspberry Juice

Pomegranate Pleasure

Watermelon Ginger Fizz

Fragrant Fruit Juice Blend

Cranberry Rhubarb Cooler

Iced Pear Juice

Sweet and Sour Strawberry Lemonade

Ruby-Red Juice Blend

Black Beauty Juice

Papaya Nectarine Juice

Cherry Coconut Juice

Razzy Rainbow Juice

Blackberry Basil Juice

Brilliant Blueberry Breakfast Blend

Kiwi Strawberry Juice Blend

Refreshing Red Berry Juice

Blessed Blood Orange Juice Blend

Sweet Lemon Lavender Juice

Sunrise Citrus Spritzer

Jicama Ginger Pear Juice

Easy Breezy Blueberry Blend

Orange Blossom Juice

MAKES 2 TO 3 SERVINGS, 8 TO 10 OUNCES EACH

Orange blossom water is nothing more than a distillation of orange blossoms. It adds a unique flavor and an appealing aroma to traditional orange juice.

4 NAVEL ORANGES, HALVED AND PEELED
1 TEASPOON ORANGE BLOSSOM WATER

1. Section the oranges as needed to fit into the feed chute of your juicer.

2. Place a pitcher or container under the spout of the juicer.

3. Feed the oranges through the juicer.

4. Stir the orange blossom water into the juice; then pour the juice into glasses and serve immediately.

5. Fresh juice may be refrigerated in an airtight container for up to 3 days.

Pineapple Apple Juice

Pineapple is an excellent source of vitamin C and also contains high levels of certain anti-inflammatory compounds like bromelain to promote joint health.

3 MEDIUM APPLES
½ PINEAPPLE, CORED AND HUSKED
½ INCH GINGERROOT

1. Trim or chop the ingredients as needed to fit into the feed chute of your juicer.

2. Place a pitcher or container under the spout of the juicer.

3. Feed the ingredients through the juicer in the order listed.

4. Stir the juice briefly; then pour it into glasses and serve immediately.

5. Fresh juice may be refrigerated in an airtight container for up to 3 days.

Cran-Raspberry Spritzer

If you're looking for a juice that's delicious as well as attractive, look no further than this spritzer. Fresh cranberries and raspberries combine for a rich color.

2 CUPS FRESH CRANBERRIES
1 MEDIUM NAVEL ORANGE, HALVED AND PEELED
1 LIME, HALVED AND PEELED
½ CUP RASPBERRIES
2 TO 3 TABLESPOONS SPARKLING WATER

1. Trim or chop the orange and lime as needed to fit into the feed chute of your juicer.

2. Place a pitcher or container under the spout of the juicer.

3. Feed the first 3 ingredients through the juicer in the order listed.

4. Divide the fresh raspberries between 2 glasses and top with ice.

5. Stir the juice briefly; then pour it into the glasses.

6. Top each glass with a splash of sparkling water to serve.

7. Fresh juice may be refrigerated in an airtight container for up to 3 days.

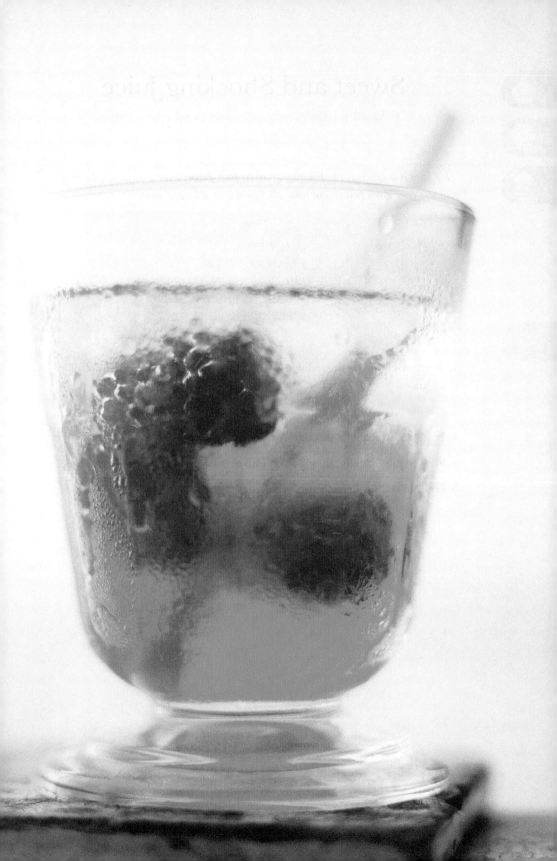

Sweet and Shocking Juice

This juice is a delicious combination of sweet fruit flavors with a surprising burst of sourness from green grapes and lime, all topped with a hint of mint.

2 KIWIS, PEELED
1 MANGO, PITTED
1 CUP SEEDLESS GREEN GRAPES
1 LIME, HALVED AND PEELED
2 TO 3 SPRIGS FRESH MINT

1. Trim or chop the ingredients as needed to fit into the feed chute of your juicer.

2. Place a pitcher or container under the spout of the juicer.

3. Feed the ingredients through the juicer in the order listed.

4. Stir the juice briefly; then pour it into glasses and serve immediately.

5. Fresh juice may be refrigerated in an airtight container for up to 3 days.

Strawberry Watermelon Juice

In this recipe the sweet flavors of strawberry and watermelon are balanced with the cool, refreshing flavor of fresh cilantro—perfect for a summer evening spent on the porch.

1 SMALL SEEDLESS WATERMELON, RIND REMOVED
2 CUPS STRAWBERRIES
¼ CUP FRESH CILANTRO LEAVES

1. Trim or chop the ingredients as needed to fit into the feed chute of your juicer.

2. Place a pitcher or container under the spout of the juicer.

3. Feed the ingredients through the juicer in the order listed.

4. Stir the juice briefly; then pour it into glasses and serve immediately.

5. Fresh juice may be refrigerated in an airtight container for up to 3 days.

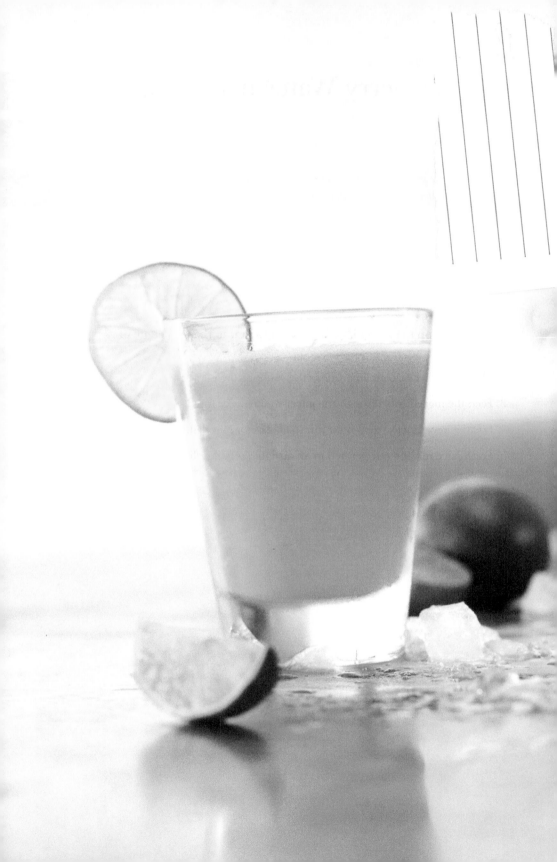

Honeyed Cantaloupe Tonic

Cantaloupe juice has a cool and refreshing flavor, not to mention a high concentration of vitamins and minerals. In this recipe, the subtle sweetness of cantaloupe is amplified by the addition of raw honey.

1 MEDIUM CANTALOUPE, RIND REMOVED
1 NAVEL ORANGE, HALVED AND PEELED
½ LIME, PEELED
2 TABLESPOONS RAW HONEY

1. Trim or chop the ingredients as needed to fit into the feed chute of your juicer.

2. Place a pitcher or container under the spout of the juicer.

3. Feed the first 3 ingredients through the juicer in the order listed.

4. Stir the honey into the juice; then pour the juice into glasses and serve immediately.

5. Fresh juice may be refrigerated in an airtight container for up to 3 days.

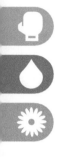

Sparkling Citrus Juice

If you're looking for a juice to put a little pep in your step, try this invigorating recipe.

1 MEDIUM GRAPEFRUIT, HALVED AND PEELED
1 BLOOD ORANGE, HALVED AND PEELED
1 NECTARINE, PITTED
½ LEMON, PEELED
2½ CUPS SPARKLING WATER, COLD

1. Trim or chop the ingredients as needed to fit into the feed chute of your juicer.

2. Place a pitcher or container under the spout of the juicer.

3. Feed the first 4 ingredients through the juicer in the order listed.

4. Stir the sparkling water into the juice; then pour the juice into glasses and serve immediately.

5. Fresh juice may be refrigerated in an airtight container for up to 3 days.

Pretty in Pink

Plums are delicious when eaten raw, but few people think to use them for juicing. They provide a number of health benefits, including protection against macular degeneration and free radical damage.

4 RED PLUMS, PITTED
1 MEDIUM PINK GRAPEFRUIT, HALVED AND PEELED
½ BUNCH OR 2 CUPS ROMAINE LETTUCE
1 POMEGRANATE

1. Trim or chop the ingredients as needed to fit into the feed chute of your juicer.

2. Place a pitcher or container under the spout of the juicer.

3. Feed the first 3 ingredients through the juicer in the order listed.

4. Juice the pomegranate by hand using a citrus juicer.

5. Stir the pomegranate juice into the plum mixture; then pour the juice into glasses and serve immediately.

6. Fresh juice may be refrigerated in an airtight container for up to 3 days.

Black Cherry Basil Blast

If you're looking for a good juice to share, this black cherry blend is just what you need. Full of flavor and pretty as a picture, it's perfect for brunch or lunch gatherings.

2¼ CUPS SLICED BLACK CHERRIES, PITTED
1 MEDIUM APPLE
½ CUP FRESH BASIL LEAVES, PACKED
⅓ CUP SPARKLING WATER

1. Reserve ¼ cup black cherries and set them aside.

2. Trim or chop the ingredients as needed to fit into the feed chute of your juicer.

3. Place a pitcher or container under the spout of the juicer.

4. Feed the first 3 ingredients through the juicer in the order listed.

5. Divide the remaining sliced cherries between 2 glasses.

6. Stir the juice briefly; then pour it into the glasses.

7. Top off each glass with sparkling water to serve.

8. Fresh juice may be refrigerated in an airtight container for up to 3 days.

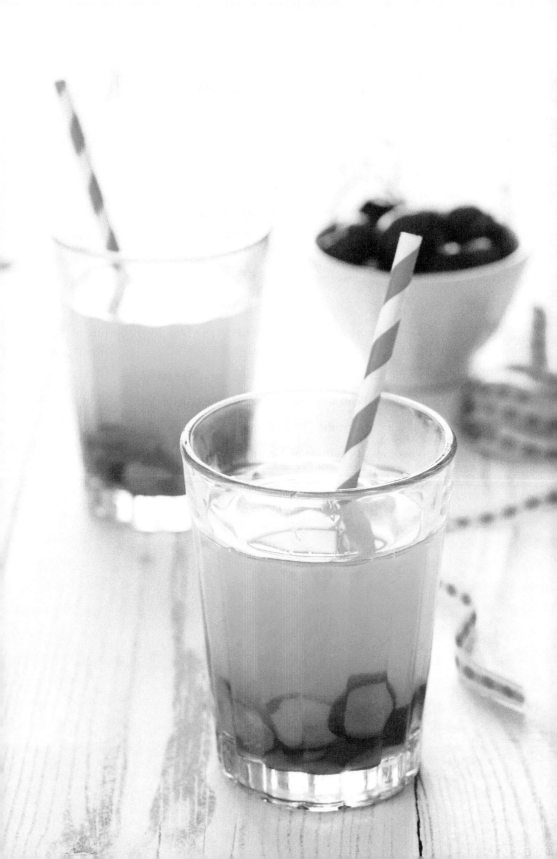

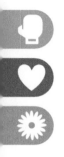

Morning Melon Wake-Up Juice

MAKES 3 TO 4 SERVINGS, 8 TO 10 OUNCES EACH

The fruit flavor of this morning melon juice will have you out of bed and on your feet in no time.

2 CUPS CHOPPED SEEDLESS WATERMELON, RIND REMOVED
½ CANTALOUPE, RIND REMOVED
½ HONEYDEW, RIND REMOVED

1. Trim or chop the ingredients as needed to fit into the feed chute of your juicer.

2. Place a pitcher or container under the spout of the juicer.

3. Feed the ingredients through the juicer in the order listed.

4. Stir the juice briefly; then pour it into glasses and serve immediately.

5. Fresh juice may be refrigerated in an airtight container for up to 3 days.

Peachy Pomegranate Juice

Though pomegranates can be tricky to deal with, they yield a delicious juice that blends well with the flavor of peach in this recipe.

4 LARGE PEACHES, PITTED
1 NAVEL ORANGE, HALVED AND PEELED
2 POMEGRANATES

1. Trim or chop the ingredients as needed to fit into the feed chute of your juicer.

2. Place a pitcher or container under the spout of the juicer.

3. Feed the peaches through the juicer and then the orange.

4. Stir the juice briefly; then pour it into glasses.

5. Juice the pomegranates by hand using a citrus juicer.

6. Add the pomegranate juice to the glasses, stir, and serve immediately.

7. Fresh juice may be refrigerated in an airtight container for up to 3 days.

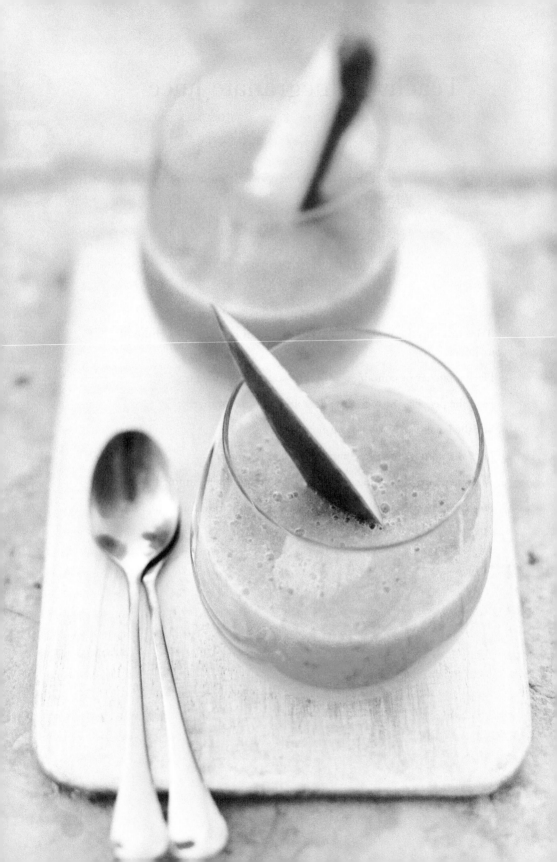

Cucumber Melon Cooler

True to its name, this recipe is the ultimate refreshing beverage to cool you down on a hot day. Full of fresh fruit flavor, it's just the thing to quench your thirst.

1 MEDIUM ENGLISH CUCUMBER
½ MEDIUM CANTALOUPE, RIND REMOVED
½ MEDIUM HONEYDEW, RIND REMOVED

1. Trim or chop the ingredients as needed to fit into the feed chute of your juicer. If desired, place a few thin slices of cucumber aside to use as a garnish.

2. Place a pitcher or container under the spout of the juicer.

3. Feed the ingredients through the juicer in the order listed.

4. Stir the juice briefly; then pour it into glasses.

5. Garnish with thin slices of cucumber (if using) to serve.

6. Fresh juice may be refrigerated in an airtight container for up to 3 days.

Cherry Berry Blast

Not only do the main ingredients in this recipe rhyme, but their flavors also work together perfectly.

2 CUPS CHERRIES, PITTED
1 CUP STRAWBERRIES
1 CUP BLACKBERRIES
PINCH OF GROUND CINNAMON

1. Place a pitcher or container under the spout of the juicer.

2. Feed the first 3 ingredients through the juicer in the order listed.

3. Add cinnamon to the juice and stir briefly.

4. Pour the juice into glasses and serve immediately.

5. Fresh juice may be refrigerated in an airtight container for up to 3 days.

Calming Tropical Juice Blend

Lavender is known for its calming properties, which is why it is often used in tea. It has also been known used as an herbal remedy for insomnia because it helps improve sleep patterns.

2 KIWIS, PEELED

1 MANGO, PITTED

1 ORANGE, HALVED AND PEELED

½ PINEAPPLE, CORED AND HUSKED

1 TO 2 TEASPOONS DRIED LAVENDER

1. Trim or chop the ingredients as needed to fit into the feed chute of your juicer.

2. Place a pitcher or container under the spout of the juicer.

3. Feed the first 4 ingredients through the juicer in the order listed.

4. Stir the dried lavender into the juice; then pour the juice into glasses and serve immediately.

5. Fresh juice may be refrigerated in an airtight container for up to 3 days.

Soothing Strawberry Juice

Mint is known not only for its unique flavor but also for its ability to relieve minor aches and pains. Combined with the sweet flavor of strawberries, that makes this recipe nearly perfect.

2 CUPS STRAWBERRIES
1 MEDIUM APPLE
2 LARGE STALKS CELERY
1 BUNCH FRESH MINT LEAVES

1. Trim or chop the ingredients as needed to fit into the feed chute of your juicer.

2. Place a pitcher or container under the spout of the juicer.

3. Feed the ingredients through the juicer in the order listed.

4. Stir the juice briefly; then pour it into glasses and serve immediately.

5. Fresh juice may be refrigerated in an airtight container for up to 3 days.

Gooseberry Goodness

Gooseberries are similar in appearance to grapes and known for their sour flavor. To combat the sourness, this recipe incorporates a sweet nectarine and honeydew.

2 CUPS GOOSEBERRIES
1 NECTARINE, PITTED
½ SMALL HONEYDEW, RIND REMOVED

1. Trim or chop the ingredients as needed to fit into the feed chute of your juicer.

2. Place a pitcher or container under the spout of the juicer.

3. Feed the ingredients through the juicer in the order listed.

4. Stir the juice briefly; then pour it into glasses and serve immediately.

5. Fresh juice may be refrigerated in an airtight container for up to 3 days.

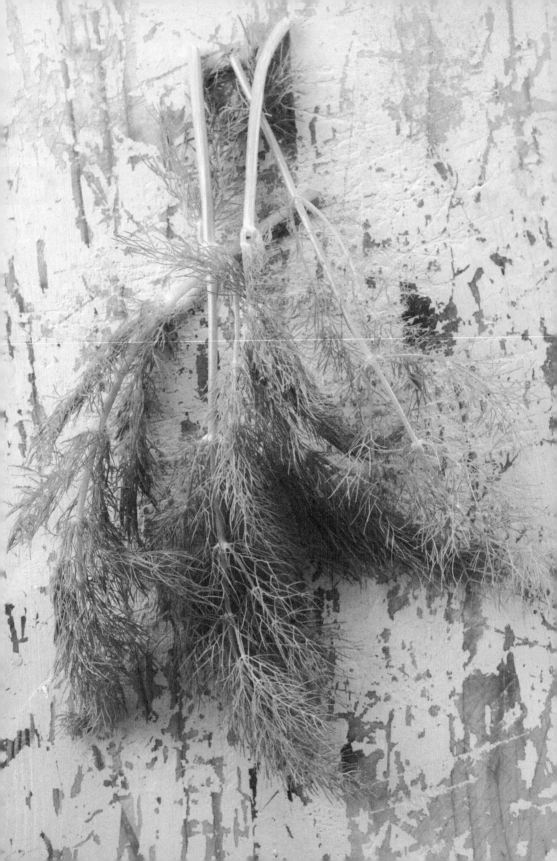

Fruity Fennel Juice Blend

This recipe combines the flavors of several different fruits and tops it all off with the crisp, refreshing taste of fennel.

2 MEDIUM PEACHES, PITTED
2 KIWIS, PEELED
1 PINT STRAWBERRIES
1 LARGE APPLE
1 SMALL BULB FENNEL

1. Trim or chop the ingredients as needed to fit into the feed chute of your juicer.

2. Place a pitcher or container under the spout of the juicer.

3. Feed the ingredients through the juicer in the order listed.

4. Stir the juice briefly; then pour it into glasses and serve immediately.

5. Fresh juice may be refrigerated in an airtight container for up to 3 days.

Kiwi Lime Spritzer

Fresh kiwis contain high concentrations of vitamin C, as do fresh limes. The flavors of these fruits, combined with the freshness of cilantro, makes for a highly refreshing drink.

4 KIWIS, PEELED

2 LIMES, HALVED AND PEELED

2 SPRIGS FRESH CILANTRO

1. Trim or chop the ingredients as needed to fit into the feed chute of your juicer.

2. Place a pitcher or container under the spout of the juicer.

3. Feed the ingredients through the juicer in the order listed.

4. Stir the juice briefly; then pour it into glasses and serve immediately.

5. Fresh juice may be refrigerated in an airtight container for up to 3 days.

Minty Melon Juice Blend

Mint is known to soothe both indigestion and inflammation. The scent alone has been shown to stimulate salivary glands, which helps improve digestion.

2 CUPS CHOPPED SEEDLESS WATERMELON, RIND REMOVED
1 SMALL CANTALOUPE, RIND REMOVED
½ SMALL HONEYDEW, RIND REMOVED
¼ BUNCH FRESH MINT LEAVES

1. Trim or chop the ingredients as needed to fit into the feed chute of your juicer.

2. Place a pitcher or container under the spout of the juicer.

3. Feed the ingredients through the juicer in the order listed.

4. Stir the juice briefly; then pour it into glasses and serve immediately.

5. Fresh juice may be refrigerated in an airtight container for up to 3 days.

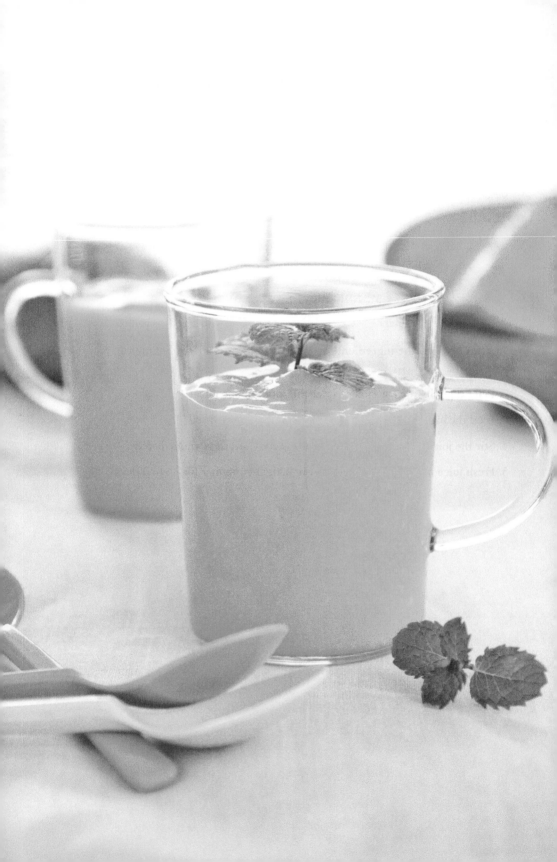

Merry Mango Juice

Combining mango with cantaloupe gives this juice a beautiful orange color.

2 MEDIUM MANGOS, PITTED
½ SMALL CANTALOUPE, RIND REMOVED
2 SPRIGS FRESH MINT, FOR GARNISH

1. Trim or chop the ingredients as needed to fit into the feed chute of your juicer.

2. Place a pitcher or container under the spout of the juicer.

3. Feed the mangos through the juicer and then the cantaloupe.

4. Stir the juice briefly; then pour it into glasses and garnish with mint to serve.

5. Fresh juice may be refrigerated in an airtight container for up to 3 days.

Lemongrass Apple Juice

Both the leaves and essential oil from the lemongrass plant are widely used in herbal remedies. This plant is beneficial for the treatment of digestive problems, high blood pressure, coughing, and rheumatism.

4 MEDIUM APPLES
1 STALK LEMONGRASS
1 SPRIG FRESH MINT
½ LEMON, PEELED

1. Trim or chop the ingredients as needed to fit into the feed chute of your juicer.

2. Place a pitcher or container under the spout of the juicer.

3. Feed the ingredients through the juicer in the order listed.

4. Stir the juice briefly; then pour it into glasses and serve immediately.

5. Fresh juice may be refrigerated in an airtight container for up to 3 days.

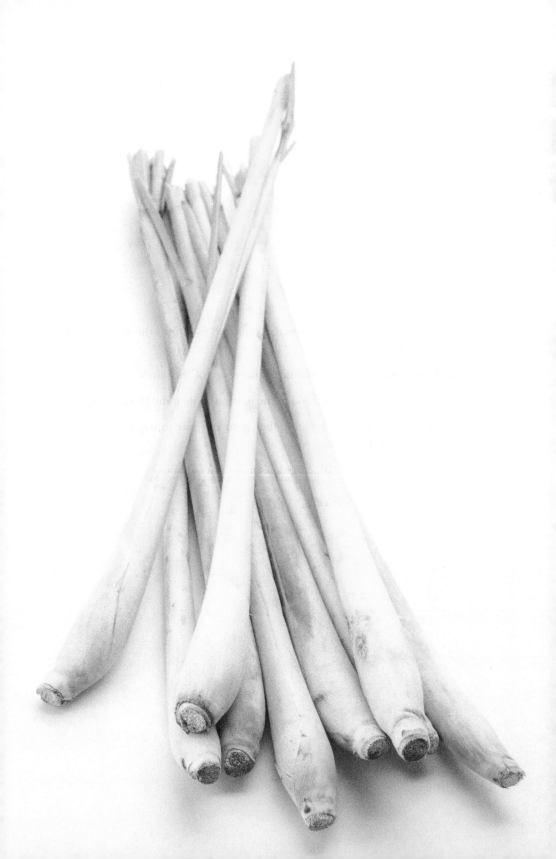

Orange Lavender Juice

This zippy juice incorporates the unique flavors of both blood oranges and lavender. What a powerful combo!

4 NAVEL ORANGES, HALVED AND PEELED
1 MEDIUM BLOOD ORANGE, HALVED AND PEELED
2 TEASPOONS DRIED LAVENDER

1. Trim or section the ingredients as needed to fit into the feed chute of your juicer.

2. Place a pitcher or container under the spout of the juicer.

3. Feed the navel oranges through the juicer and then the blood orange.

4. Stir the lavender into the juice; then pour the juice into glasses and serve immediately.

5. Fresh juice may be refrigerated in an airtight container for up to 3 days.

Passion Fruit Crush

Passion fruit contains high levels of both vitamin C and vitamin A. It's also high in potassium, which helps regulate blood pressure.

2 PASSION FRUIT
1 MEDIUM APPLE
1 MEDIUM NAVEL ORANGE, HALVED AND PEELED

1. Trim or chop the ingredients as needed to fit into the feed chute of your juicer.

2. Place a pitcher or container under the spout of the juicer.

3. Feed the ingredients through the juicer in the order listed.

4. Stir the juice briefly; then pour it into glasses and serve immediately.

5. Fresh juice may be refrigerated in an airtight container for up to 3 days.

Very Berry Juice Blend

The beauty of this recipe is that you can mix and match whatever berries you have on hand. You can even play with the proportions to turn up your favorite flavors.

1 CUP BLACKBERRIES
1 CUP RASPBERRIES
1 CUP STRAWBERRIES
½ CUP GOOSEBERRIES

1. Place a pitcher or container under the spout of the juicer.

2. Feed the ingredients through the juicer in the order listed.

3. Stir the juice briefly; then pour it into glasses and serve immediately.

4. Fresh juice may be refrigerated in an airtight container for up to 3 days.

Royal-Red Raspberry Juice

Raspberries may be the star of this juice, but don't forget the persimmon. Persimmon is a low-calorie fruit that is high in dietary fiber, antioxidants, and powerful phytonutrients.

2 CUPS RASPBERRIES
1 MEDIUM PERSIMMON
1 BLOOD ORANGE, HALVED AND PEELED
PINCH OF GROUND NUTMEG

1. Trim or chop the ingredients as needed to fit into the feed chute of your juicer.

2. Place a pitcher or container under the spout of the juicer.

3. Feed the first 3 ingredients through the juicer in the order listed.

4. Stir the nutmeg into the juice; then pour the juice into glasses and serve immediately.

5. Fresh juice may be refrigerated in an airtight container for up to 3 days.

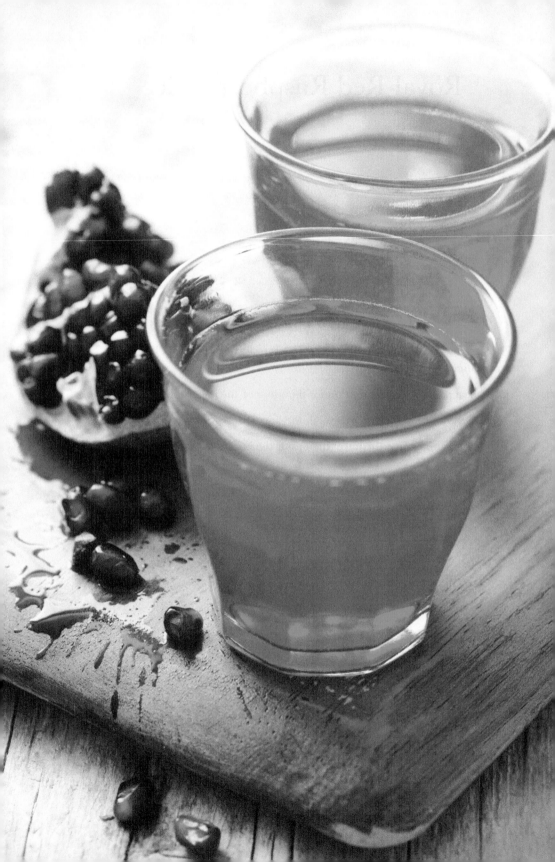

Pomegranate Pleasure

Though pomegranates have a delicious, unique flavor, they don't yield a lot of juice. Combining pomegranates with other fruits increases the yield of the recipe.

1 MEDIUM NAVEL ORANGE, HALVED AND PEELED
1 SMALL LIME, HALVED AND PEELED
4 MEDIUM POMEGRANATES

1. Place a pitcher or container under the spout of the juicer.

2. Feed the orange and lime through the juicer.

3. Juice the pomegranates by hand using a citrus juicer.

4. Stir the pomegranate juice into the orange and lime juice; then pour it into glasses and serve immediately.

5. Fresh juice may be refrigerated in an airtight container for up to 3 days.

Watermelon Ginger Fizz

If you're looking for a refreshing summertime drink, this watermelon ginger fizz may be right for you. Topping each glass with a splash of sparkling water helps give this recipe its "fizz."

1 SMALL SEEDLESS WATERMELON, RIND REMOVED
1 INCH GINGERROOT
SPARKLING WATER TO SERVE

1. Trim or chop the ingredients as needed to fit into the feed chute of your juicer.

2. Place a pitcher or container under the spout of the juicer.

3. Feed the watermelon through the juicer and then the ginger.

4. Stir the juice briefly; then pour it into glasses.

5. Top each glass with a splash of sparkling water to serve.

6. Fresh juice may be refrigerated in an airtight container for up to 3 days.

Fragrant Fruit Juice Blend

Though the fruit flavors of this juice blend are not to be forgotten, the real stars are the fragrant herbs and spices that give it such an appealing aroma.

3 NECTARINES, PITTED
2 MEDIUM PEACHES, PITTED
1 APRICOT, PITTED
1 TEASPOON DRIED LAVENDER
1 TEASPOON DRIED CORIANDER
PINCH OF GROUND TARRAGON

1. Trim or chop the ingredients as needed to fit into the feed chute of your juicer.

2. Place a pitcher or container under the spout of the juicer.

3. Feed the first 3 ingredients through the juicer in the order listed.

4. Add lavender, coriander, and tarragon to juice, and stir briefly.

5. Pour the juice into the glasses and serve immediately.

6. Fresh juice may be refrigerated in an airtight container for up to 3 days.

Cranberry Rhubarb Cooler

Though it looks remarkably similar to celery, rhubarb is actually a fruit. Rhubarb is incredibly high in fiber, which is generally a good thing. But it can make it tough for your body to digest the other nutrients, because it's working so hard to break down the fiber. That's where juicing comes in handy.

2 CUPS FRESH CRANBERRIES
2 LARGE STALKS RHUBARB
2 MEDIUM PEARS
1 SPRIG FRESH MINT
½ LEMON, PEELED

1. Trim or chop the ingredients as needed to fit into the feed chute of your juicer.

2. Place a pitcher or container under the spout of the juicer.

3. Feed the ingredients through the juicer in the order listed.

4. Stir the juice briefly; then pour it into glasses and serve immediately.

5. Fresh juice may be refrigerated in an airtight container for up to 3 days.

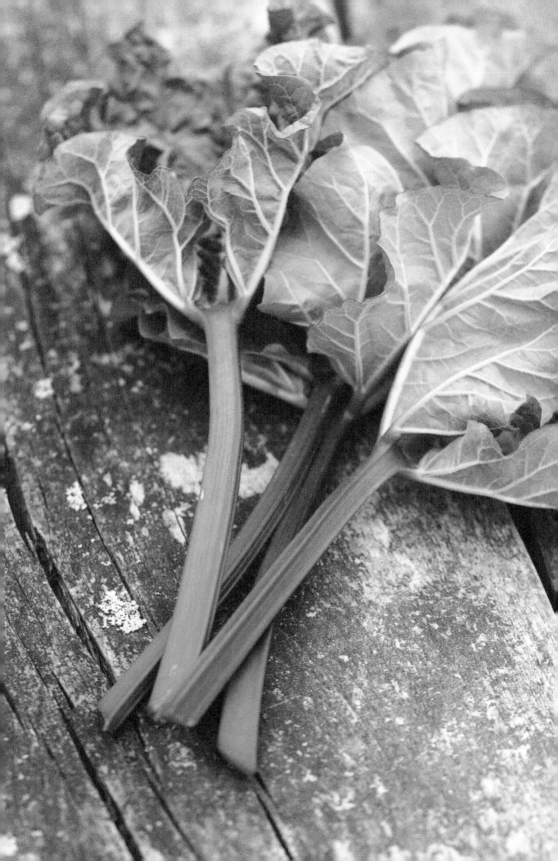

Iced Pear Juice

This iced juice is the perfect recipe to enjoy on a hot day. Made with freshly juiced pears and iced coconut water, it's truly refreshing.

4 MEDIUM PEARS
2½ CUPS COCONUT WATER
ICE CUBES TO SERVE

1. Trim or chop the pears as needed to fit into the feed chute of your juicer.

2. Place a pitcher or container under the spout of the juicer.

3. Feed the pears through the juicer.

4. Stir the coconut water into the pear juice, and pour it into glasses.

5. Add ice cubes to serve.

6. Fresh juice may be refrigerated in an airtight container for up to 3 days.

Sweet and Sour
Strawberry Lemonade

This recipe can easily be customized to suit your tastes. If you prefer your lemonade on the sweeter side, add an extra handful of strawberries. If you like sour lemonade, add extra lemon or lime.

4 TO 6 LEMONS, HALVED AND PEELED
1 CUP STRAWBERRIES
½ SMALL LIME, PEELED
WATER FOR DILUTING (OPTIONAL)

1. Trim or chop the ingredients as needed to fit into the feed chute of your juicer.

2. Place a pitcher or container under the spout of the juicer.

3. Feed the first 3 ingredients through the juicer in the order listed.

4. Stir the juice briefly; then pour it into glasses.

5. Dilute the juice with water if the lemon flavor is too strong for your taste.

6. Fresh juice may be refrigerated in an airtight container for up to 3 days.

Ruby-Red Juice Blend

This ruby-red juice uses the citrusy flavor of red grapefruit as a foundation, with hints of cherry, peach, and plum.

2 MEDIUM RED GRAPEFRUIT, HALVED AND PEELED
2 SMALL PLUMS, PITTED
1 MEDIUM PEACH, PITTED
1 CUP CHERRIES, PITTED

1. Trim or chop the ingredients as needed to fit into the feed chute of your juicer.

2. Place a pitcher or container under the spout of the juicer.

3. Feed the ingredients through the juicer in the order listed.

4. Stir the juice briefly; then pour it into glasses and serve immediately.

5. Fresh juice may be refrigerated in an airtight container for up to 3 days.

Black Beauty Juice

Blackberries are an excellent source of antioxidants, including ellagic acid, which has been shown to help repair sun-damaged skin. They also contain vitamin C, which may help reduce the appearance of wrinkles.

1 PINT BLACKBERRIES
2 MEDIUM APPLES
½ SMALL LEMON, PEELED

1. Trim or chop the ingredients as needed to fit into the feed chute of your juicer.

2. Place a pitcher or container under the spout of the juicer.

3. Feed the ingredients through the juicer in the order listed.

4. Stir the juice briefly; then pour it into glasses and serve immediately.

5. Fresh juice may be refrigerated in an airtight container for up to 3 days.

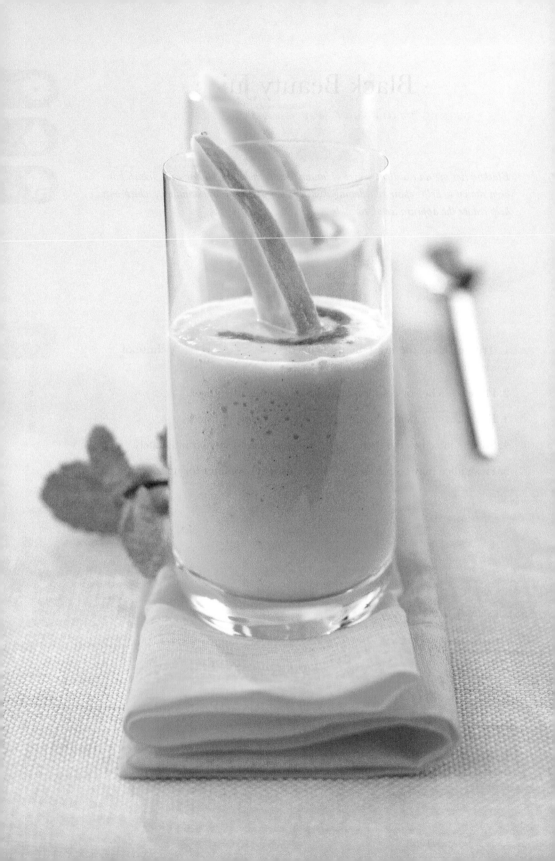

Papaya Nectarine Juice

Papaya is a sweet fruit with a soft consistency and exotic flavor. It provides a number of health benefits, including supporting the immune system and helping protect against heart disease and macular degeneration.

2 MEDIUM PAPAYAS, SEEDED
2 MEDIUM NECTARINES, PITTED
1 CUP CHOPPED SEEDLESS WATERMELON, RIND REMOVED
2 THIN SLICES PAPAYA FOR GARNISH

1. Trim or chop the ingredients as needed to fit into the feed chute of your juicer.

2. Place a pitcher or container under the spout of the juicer.

3. Feed the first 3 ingredients through the juicer in the order listed.

4. Stir the juice briefly; then pour it into glasses.

5. Garnish with slices of papaya to serve.

6. Fresh juice may be refrigerated in an airtight container for up to 3 days.

Cherry Coconut Juice

Cherry and coconut are two flavors that you might not typically picture together. After trying this recipe, however, you might think these two are a match made in heaven.

1 PINT CHERRIES, PITTED
2 TO 3 CUPS COLD COCONUT WATER

1. Place a pitcher or container under the spout of the juicer.

2. Feed the cherries through the juicer.

3. Stir the coconut water into the juice; then pour the juice into glasses and serve immediately.

4. Fresh juice may be refrigerated in an airtight container for up to 3 days.

Razzy Rainbow Juice

This recipe is aptly named because its ingredients represent nearly all of the colors of the rainbow.

2 KIWIS, PEELED
2 PLUMS, PITTED
1 CUP RASPBERRIES
1 HANDFUL KUMQUATS
½ CUP BLUEBERRIES
½ SMALL LEMON, PEELED

1. Trim or chop the ingredients as needed to fit into the feed chute of your juicer.

2. Place a pitcher or container under the spout of the juicer.

3. Feed the ingredients through the juicer in the order listed.

4. Stir the juice briefly; then pour it into glasses and serve immediately.

5. Fresh juice may be refrigerated in an airtight container for up to 3 days.

Blackberry Basil Juice

Blackberries give this juice a deep, blue-black color as well as a boost of healthful vitamins and minerals. In fact, the color of these berries is related to the reason that they have one of the highest concentrations of antioxidants of any fruit.

2 PINTS BLACKBERRIES
½ CUP FRESH BASIL LEAVES, PACKED
½ LIME, PEELED

1. Place a pitcher or container under the spout of the juicer.

2. Feed the ingredients through the juicer in the order listed.

3. Stir the juice briefly; then pour it into glasses and serve immediately.

4. Fresh juice may be refrigerated in an airtight container for up to 3 days.

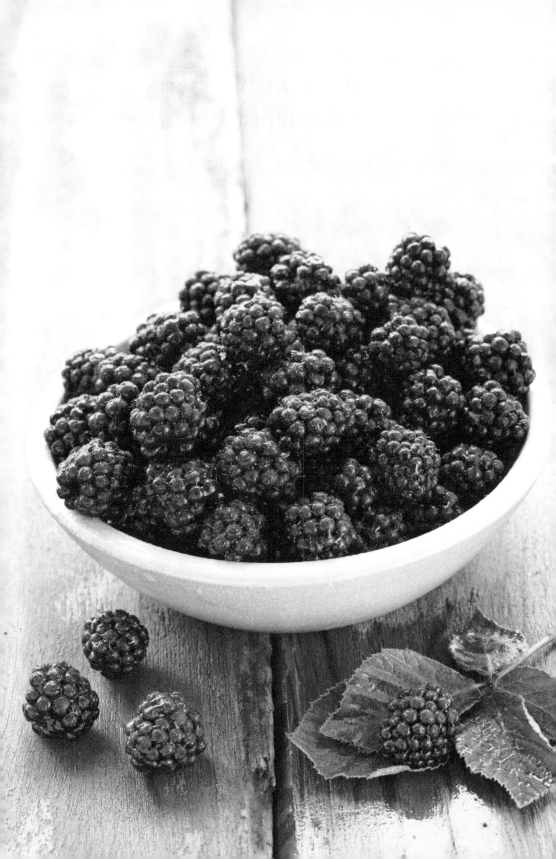

Brilliant Blueberry
Breakfast Blend

This recipe is designed to wake you up with a burst of flavor and natural energy—just what you need to start your day.

1 CUP BLUEBERRIES
2 KIWIS, PEELED
½ BUNCH OR 1 CUP ROMAINE LETTUCE
1 SPRIG FRESH DILL

1. Trim or chop the ingredients as needed to fit into the feed chute of your juicer.

2. Place a pitcher or container under the spout of the juicer.

3. Feed the ingredients through the juicer in the order listed.

4. Stir the juice briefly; then pour it into glasses and serve immediately.

5. Fresh juice may be refrigerated in an airtight container for up to 3 days.

Kiwi Strawberry Juice Blend

MAKES 2 SERVINGS, 8 TO 10 OUNCES EACH

The classic blend of strawberries and kiwis has never tasted as good as it does in this simple recipe. You have to try it yourself and see.

2 CUPS STRAWBERRIES
3 KIWIS, PEELED

1. Trim or chop the ingredients as needed to fit into the feed chute of your juicer.

2. Place a pitcher or container under the spout of the juicer.

3. Feed the ingredients through the juicer in the order listed.

4. Stir the juice briefly; then pour it into glasses and serve immediately.

5. Fresh juice may be refrigerated in an airtight container for up to 3 days.

Refreshing Red Berry Juice

Berries are an excellent source of vitamins and minerals, including vitamin C, potassium, calcium, and iron.

2 CUPS STRAWBERRIES
1 CUP RASPBERRIES
1 CUP GOOSEBERRIES
1 CUP SEEDLESS RED GRAPES

1. Place a pitcher or container under the spout of the juicer.

2. Feed the ingredients through the juicer in the order listed.

3. Stir the juice briefly; then pour it into glasses and serve immediately.

4. Fresh juice may be refrigerated in an airtight container for up to 3 days.

Blessed Blood Orange Juice Blend

Given the unique flavors of both blood oranges and kumquats, this recipe is sure to surprise and satisfy your taste buds.

4 BLOOD ORANGES, HALVED AND PEELED
2 LARGE STALKS CELERY
1 HANDFUL KUMQUATS

1. Trim or chop the ingredients as needed to fit into the feed chute of your juicer.

2. Place a pitcher or container under the spout of the juicer.

3. Feed the ingredients through the juicer in the order listed.

4. Stir the juice briefly; then pour it into glasses and serve immediately.

5. Fresh juice may be refrigerated in an airtight container for up to 3 days.

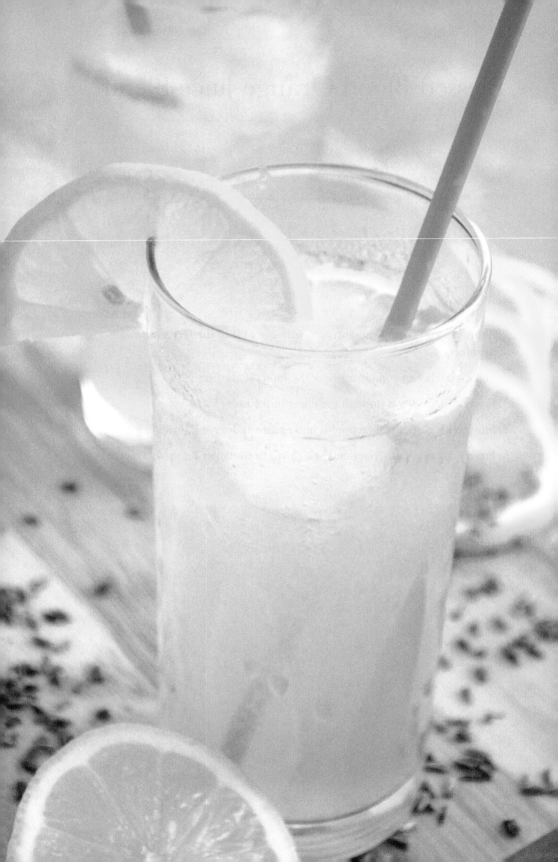

Sweet Lemon Lavender Juice

Similar to traditional lemonade, this recipe is unique in that it uses dried lavender. Lavender gives this recipe more than a hint of flavor—it also adds a calming aroma.

2 MEDIUM APPLES
2 MEDIUM LEMONS, HALVED AND PEELED
2 CUPS WATER
2 TEASPOONS DRIED LAVENDER

1. Trim or chop the apples and lemons as needed to fit into the feed chute of your juicer.

2. Place a pitcher or container under the spout of the juicer.

3. Feed the apples through the juicer and then the lemons.

4. Stir the water and lavender into the juice; then pour the juice into glasses and serve.

5. Fresh juice may be refrigerated in an airtight container for up to 3 days.

Sunrise Citrus Spritzer

The light, citrusy flavor of this recipe is just the thing you need to wake you up in the morning. And don't forget about all of that vitamin C.

2 MEDIUM GRAPEFRUITS, HALVED AND PEELED
2 NECTARINES, PITTED
1 NAVEL ORANGE, HALVED AND PEELED
½ LEMON, PEELED

1. Trim or chop the ingredients as needed to fit into the feed chute of your juicer.

2. Place a pitcher or container under the spout of the juicer.

3. Feed the ingredients through the juicer in the order listed.

4. Stir the juice briefly; then pour it into glasses and serve immediately.

5. Fresh juice may be refrigerated in an airtight container for up to 3 days.

Jicama Ginger Pear Juice

Jicama is a very low-calorie food known for its subtle flavor and crunch. In this recipe it's the perfect backdrop to highlight the flavors of pear and ginger.

2 PEARS

1 JICAMA, PEELED

½ INCH GINGERROOT

1 TABLESPOON GROUND HEMP SEED

1. Trim or chop the ingredients as needed to fit into the feed chute of your juicer.

2. Place a pitcher or container under the spout of the juicer.

3. Feed the first 3 ingredients through the juicer in the order listed.

4. Stir the ground hemp seed into the juice; then pour the juice into glasses and serve immediately.

5. Fresh juice may be refrigerated in an airtight container for up to 3 days.

Easy Breezy Blueberry Blend

Blueberries are an excellent source of antioxidants, which help repair cellular damage caused by free radicals. Take advantage of your local farmers' market, or go out and pick your own blueberries for this recipe.

2 CUPS BLUEBERRIES
1 CUP CHOPPED SEEDLESS WATERMELON, RIND REMOVED
1 LIME, HALVED AND PEELED
2 SPRIGS FRESH PARSLEY

1. Place a pitcher or container under the spout of the juicer.

2. Feed the ingredients through the juicer in the order listed.

3. Stir the juice briefly; then pour it into glasses and serve immediately.

4. Fresh juice may be refrigerated in an airtight container for up to 3 days.

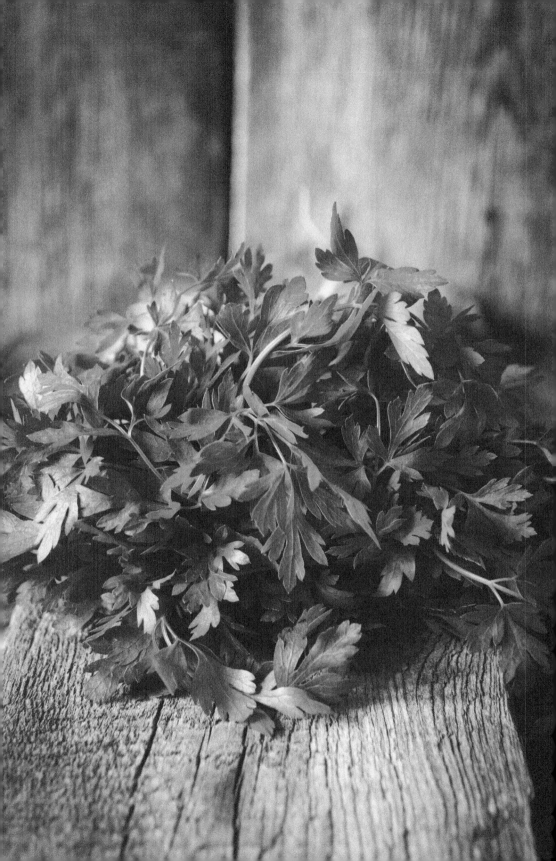

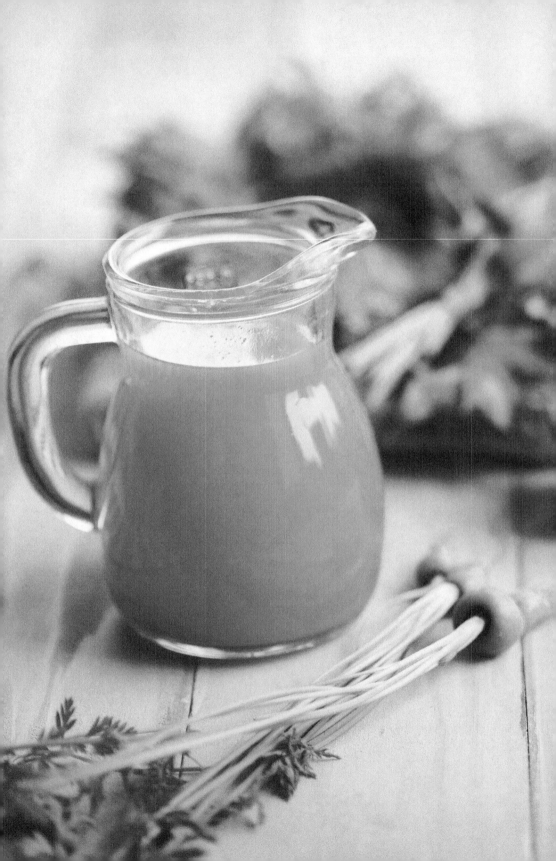

CHAPTER FIFTEEN

60 Vegetable Juices

Refreshing Juice Booster

Cool and Calming Celery Cleanse

Tomato Gazpacho Juice

Cabbage Wheatgrass Tonic

Green Pepper Ginseng Juice Blend

Purple Parsnip Juice

Tossed Salad Green Tonic

Red Cabbage Fennel Booster

Tomato and Spinach Juice

Raspberry Radish Juice

Fresh Start Detox Juice Blend

Carrot Celery Juice

Kick-Start Carrot Juice Blend

Zesty Zucchini Juice

Swiss Chard Strawberry Juice Blend

Sweet Spinach and Celery Juice

Asparagus Parsley Power Juice

Cleansing Cauliflower Carrot Juice

Beauty-Boosting Brussels Sprouts Juice

Skin-Clearing Celery Juice

Ginger Vegetable Juice Blend

Berry Beet Juice Blend

Antiaging Juice Booster

Peachy Parsley Juice

Lovely Lime Cilantro Blend

Just Plain Green Juice

Berry Basil Blusher

Green Dream Juice Blend

Sweet Swiss Chard Juice

Sweet Potato Protein Spritzer

Sweet Pea Power-Up Juice

Tasty Tomato Turnip Juice

Beautiful Broccoli Juice Blend

Dandy Dandelion Green Juice

Kale Cabbage Juice

Turnip Celery Juicer

Radish Rutabaga Juice Blend

Brilliant Brussels Sprouts Juice

Blueberry Beetroot Booster

Immune-Boosting Blast

Brain Power Beet Juice Blend

Avocado Asparagus Juice

Spinach Cucumber Celery Juice

Protein-Packed Juice Blend

Fennel Apple Juice Booster

Green Machine Juice Blend

Wrinkle-Reducing Cucumber Juice

Green Carrot Broccoli Juice

Wonderful Weight-Loss Juice

Hearty Beet and Dandelion Green Juice

Awesome Arugula Tonic

Sweet Red Pepper Broccoli Juice

Tasty Turnip Green Juice

Rockin' Red Pepper Juice

Cool Celery Limeade

Carrot Orange Ginger Juice

Homegrown Green Juice

Three-B Juice Blend

Green Bean Sprout Power Juice

Kickin' Kale Collard Green Juice

Refreshing Juice Booster

Romaine lettuce is an excellent energy-boosting vegetable that, combined with the tangy flavor of fresh lime, makes this juice incredibly refreshing. Enjoy it in the morning to wake yourself up or sip it in the afternoon to keep yourself powered-up until dinner.

2 LARGE CARROTS
2 LARGE LEAVES ROMAINE LETTUCE
1 LARGE STALK CELERY
½ SMALL ZUCCHINI
½ LIME, PEELED

1. Trim or chop the ingredients as needed to fit into the feed chute of your juicer.

2. Place a pitcher or container under the spout of the juicer.

3. Feed the ingredients through the juicer in the order listed.

4. Stir the juice briefly; then pour it into glasses and serve immediately.

5. Fresh juice may be refrigerated in an airtight container for up to 3 days.

Cool and Calming Celery Cleanse

In this recipe, the crisp peppery flavor of celery combines perfectly with the subtle sweetness of green grapes. A few sprigs of cilantro give this juice a coolness that refreshes as it cleanses.

3 LARGE CARROTS
1 LARGE STALK CELERY
1 CUP GREEN SEEDLESS GRAPES
3 TO 4 SPRIGS FRESH CILANTRO

1. Trim or chop the ingredients as needed to fit into the feed chute of your juicer.

2. Place a pitcher or container under the spout of the juicer.

3. Feed the ingredients through the juicer in the order listed.

4. Stir the juice briefly; then pour it into a glass and serve immediately.

5. Fresh juice may be refrigerated in an airtight container for up to 3 days.

Tomato Gazpacho Juice

Gazpacho is a summer soup traditionally served cold. In this recipe you get all of the flavor of fresh, raw vegetables with a hint of heat from cayenne pepper.

2 MEDIUM ROMA TOMATOES
2 SCALLIONS
1 SMALL SEEDLESS CUCUMBER
3 TO 4 FRESH BASIL LEAVES
1 GARLIC CLOVE, PEELED
PINCH OF CAYENNE PEPPER
PINCH OF SEA SALT

1. Trim or chop the ingredients as needed to fit into the feed chute of your juicer.

2. Place a pitcher or container under the spout of the juicer.

3. Feed the first 5 ingredients through the juicer in the order listed.

4. Stir the juice briefly; then pour it into glasses.

5. Stir in the cayenne pepper and sea salt; then serve immediately.

6. Fresh juice may be refrigerated in an airtight container for up to 3 days.

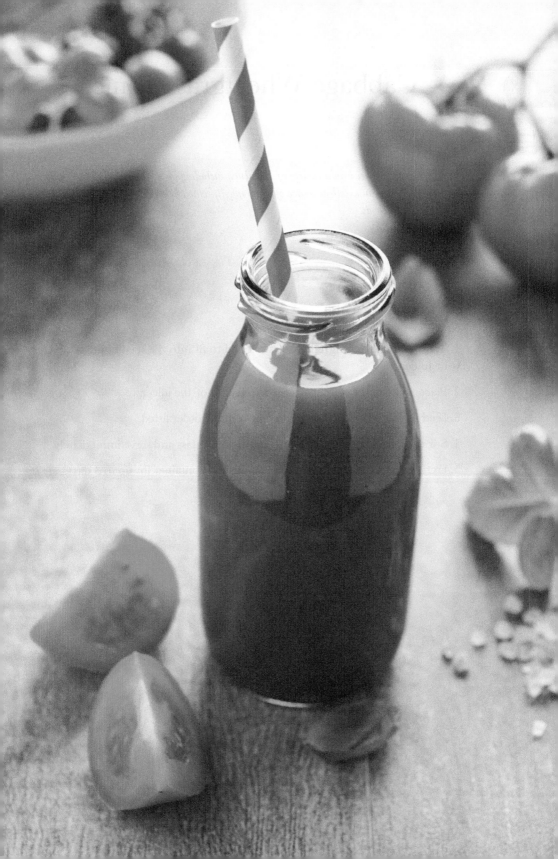

Cabbage Wheatgrass Tonic

Fresh wheatgrass is rich in a variety of nutrients, including amino acids, vitamins, and enzymes. It's also an excellent source of chlorophyll, which helps to oxygenate the blood and detoxify the body.

1 CUP COARSELY CHOPPED GREEN CABBAGE
½ CUP WHEATGRASS
½ LEMON, PEELED

1. Trim or chop the ingredients as needed to fit into the feed chute of your juicer.

2. Place a pitcher or container under the spout of the juicer.

3. Feed the ingredients through the juicer in the order listed.

4. Stir the juice briefly; then pour it into a small glass and serve immediately.

5. Fresh juice may be refrigerated in an airtight container for up to 3 days.

Green Pepper Ginseng Juice Blend

Ginseng is a root that has long been used in Asia and North America in herbal remedies. It has been found to improve immune system health, particularly in reducing the risk for and severity of colds.

2 MEDIUM GREEN BELL PEPPERS
1 CUP FRESH PUMPKIN, CHOPPED, RIND REMOVED
1 LARGE PEACH, PITTED
½ CUP BABY SPINACH, PACKED
1 TEASPOON GINSENG POWDER

1. Trim or chop the ingredients as needed to fit into the feed chute of your juicer.

2. Place a pitcher or container under the spout of the juicer.

3. Feed the first 4 ingredients through the juicer in the order listed.

4. Stir the ginseng powder into the juice; then pour the juice into glasses and serve immediately.

5. Fresh juice may be refrigerated in an airtight container for up to 3 days.

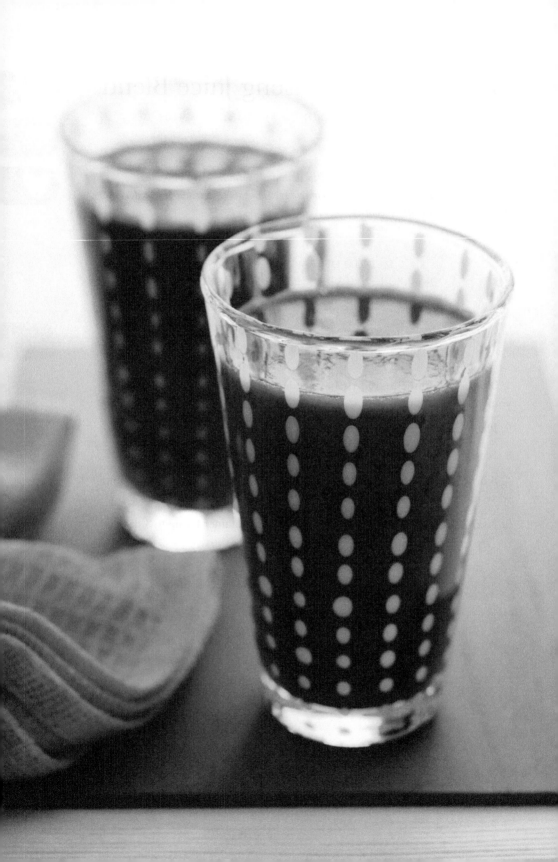

Purple Parsnip Juice

Parsnips may not contain a great deal of juice, but the concoction that results from feeding these vegetables through the juicer is sweet and creamy. Combined with apples and blueberries, this juice is a refreshing treat.

2 PARSNIPS
1 MEDIUM APPLE
½ CUP BLUEBERRIES
¼ BUNCH FRESH PARSLEY

1. Trim or chop the ingredients as needed to fit into the feed chute of your juicer.

2. Place a pitcher or container under the spout of the juicer.

3. Feed the ingredients through the juicer in the order listed.

4. Stir the juice briefly; then pour it into glasses and serve immediately.

5. Fresh juice may be refrigerated in an airtight container for up to 3 days.

Tossed Salad Green Tonic

If you're looking for a cool and refreshing meal but don't have time to sit down and eat, this tonic is perfect for you. You get all the goodness of a heaping bowl of greens without the work of chewing!

1 CUP ARUGULA, PACKED

1 CUP BABY SPINACH, PACKED

4 SMALL RADISHES

1 SMALL CUCUMBER

1 SMALL CARROT

1 LARGE APPLE

1. Trim or chop the ingredients as needed to fit into the feed chute of your juicer.

2. Place a pitcher or container under the spout of the juicer.

3. Feed the ingredients through the juicer in the order listed.

4. Stir the juice briefly; then pour it into glasses and serve immediately.

5. Fresh juice may be refrigerated in an airtight container for up to 3 days.

Red Cabbage Fennel Booster

Fennel has a crunchy texture and a sweet, refreshing flavor. It also offers a number of health benefits, including antioxidant protection, immune support, and improved colon health.

2 SMALL FENNEL BULBS
2 MEDIUM APPLES
½ SMALL BUNCH OR 1 CUP CURLY KALE
½ SMALL RED CABBAGE
½ LEMON, PEELED

1. Trim or chop the ingredients as needed to fit into the feed chute of your juicer.

2. Place a pitcher or container under the spout of the juicer.

3. Feed the ingredients through the juicer in the order listed.

4. Stir the juice briefly; then pour it into glasses and serve immediately.

5. Fresh juice may be refrigerated in an airtight container for up to 3 days.

Tomato and Spinach Juice

MAKES 3 TO 4 SERVINGS, 8 TO 10 OUNCES EACH

Heirloom tomatoes come in a variety of shapes and colors, from small red tomatoes to large yellow, green, and even purple tomatoes. These tomatoes are loaded with health benefits as well as flavor.

1 BUNCH OR 2 CUPS SPINACH LEAVES
2 LARGE HEIRLOOM TOMATOES
½ LEMON, PEELED

1. Trim or chop the ingredients as needed to fit into the feed chute of your juicer.

2. Place a pitcher or container under the spout of the juicer.

3. Feed the ingredients through the juicer in the order listed.

4. Stir the juice briefly; then pour it into glasses and serve immediately.

5. Fresh juice may be refrigerated in an airtight container for up to 3 days.

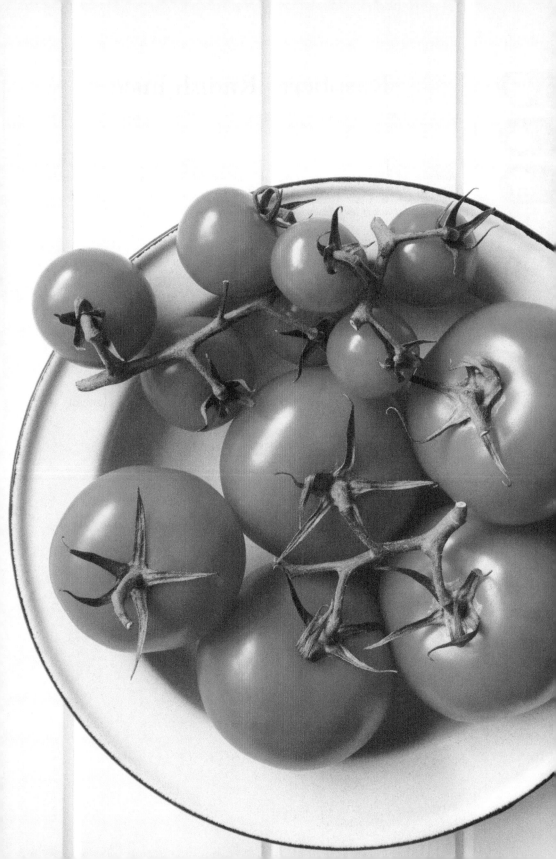

Raspberry Radish Juice

Radishes are a type of cruciferous vegetable that are rich in a variety of vitamins and minerals. The greens of radishes are actually richer in nutrients than the vegetables themselves, which is why they're included in this recipe.

6 MEDIUM RADISHES, GREENS INCLUDED
2 LARGE LEAVES DANDELION GREENS
1 CUP RASPBERRIES
1 STALK CELERY
1 MEDIUM APPLE
1 GARLIC CLOVE, PEELED

1. Trim or chop the ingredients as needed to fit into the feed chute of your juicer.

2. Place a pitcher or container under the spout of the juicer.

3. Feed the ingredients through the juicer in the order listed.

4. Stir the juice briefly; then pour it into glasses and serve immediately.

5. Fresh juice may be refrigerated in an airtight container for up to 3 days.

Fresh Start Detox Juice Blend

All the ingredients in this recipe are known for their detoxifying properties. If you're looking for the perfect recipe to start a juice cleanse, or simply want to boost your body's natural detox abilities, try this juice blend.

2 CUPS CHOPPED DANDELION GREENS
1 LARGE STALK CELERY
1 LARGE PARSNIP
3 TO 4 SPRIGS FRESH PARSLEY
½ LEMON, PEELED
½ INCH GINGERROOT

219

1. Trim or chop the ingredients as needed to fit into the feed chute of your juicer.

2. Place a pitcher or container under the spout of the juicer.

3. Feed the ingredients through the juicer in the order listed.

4. Stir the juice briefly; then pour it into glasses and serve immediately.

5. Fresh juice may be refrigerated in an airtight container for up to 3 days.

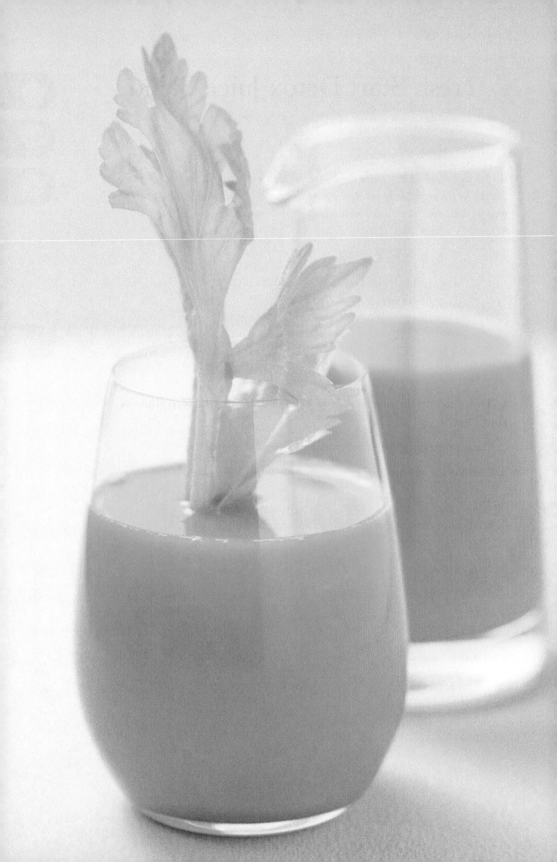

Carrot Celery Juice

Not only are carrots one of the most readily available vegetables in the food market but they're also an excellent source of vitamins and minerals. Carrots are loaded with beta-carotene and carotenoids, which help prevent cancer and reduce the risk of macular degeneration.

6 LARGE CARROTS
4 LARGE STALKS CELERY, GREENS INCLUDED
1 MEDIUM BARTLETT PEAR
¼ BUNCH FRESH PARSLEY

1. Trim or chop the ingredients as needed to fit into the feed chute of your juicer.

2. Place a pitcher or container under the spout of the juicer.

3. Feed the ingredients through the juicer in the order listed.

4. Stir the juice briefly; then pour it into glasses and serve immediately.

5. Fresh juice may be refrigerated in an airtight container for up to 3 days.

221

60 VEGETABLE JUICES

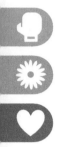

Kick-Start Carrot Juice Blend

MAKES 2 SERVINGS, 8 TO 10 OUNCES EACH

This recipe is just what you need to kick-start your day. Packed with vitamins and minerals, this juice blend also includes the protein power of dried spirulina powder.

3 LARGE CARROTS
1 MEDIUM APRICOT, PITTED
1 CUP BABY SPINACH LEAVES
½ LEMON, PEELED
1 TABLESPOON SPIRULINA POWDER

1. Trim or chop the ingredients as needed to fit into the feed chute of your juicer.

2. Place a pitcher or container under the spout of the juicer.

3. Feed the first 4 ingredients through the juicer in the order listed.

4. Stir the spirulina powder into the juice; then pour the juice into glasses and serve immediately.

5. Fresh juice may be refrigerated in an airtight container for up to 3 days.

Zesty Zucchini Juice

Zucchini is an excellent source of iron, manganese, and vitamin C. It has also been linked to reducing the risk for cardiovascular disease, which, when combined with the heart-healing power of kale, makes this recipe incredibly heart-healthful.

1 MEDIUM ZUCCHINI
1 MEDIUM BEET, GREENS INCLUDED
1 CUP CHOPPED KALE
1 SMALL SCALLION
1 SMALL LIME, HALVED AND PEELED

1. Trim or chop the ingredients as needed to fit into the feed chute of your juicer.

2. Place a pitcher or container under the spout of the juicer.

3. Feed the ingredients through the juicer in the order listed.

4. Stir the juice briefly; then pour it into glasses and serve immediately.

5. Fresh juice may be refrigerated in an airtight container for up to 3 days.

Swiss Chard Strawberry Juice Blend

Swiss chard is a leafy green vegetable known for its high concentration of vitamins and minerals. It's rich in dietary fiber and contains high levels of vitamins A, C, and K.

1 BUNCH OR 2 CUPS SWISS CHARD
1 CUP STRAWBERRIES
1 SMALL CUCUMBER
1 SMALL SCALLION
3 TO 4 SPRIGS FRESH DILL

1. Trim or chop the ingredients as needed to fit into the feed chute of your juicer.

2. Place a pitcher or container under the spout of the juicer.

3. Feed the ingredients through the juicer in the order listed.

4. Stir the juice briefly; then pour it into glasses and serve immediately.

5. Fresh juice may be refrigerated in an airtight container for up to 3 days.

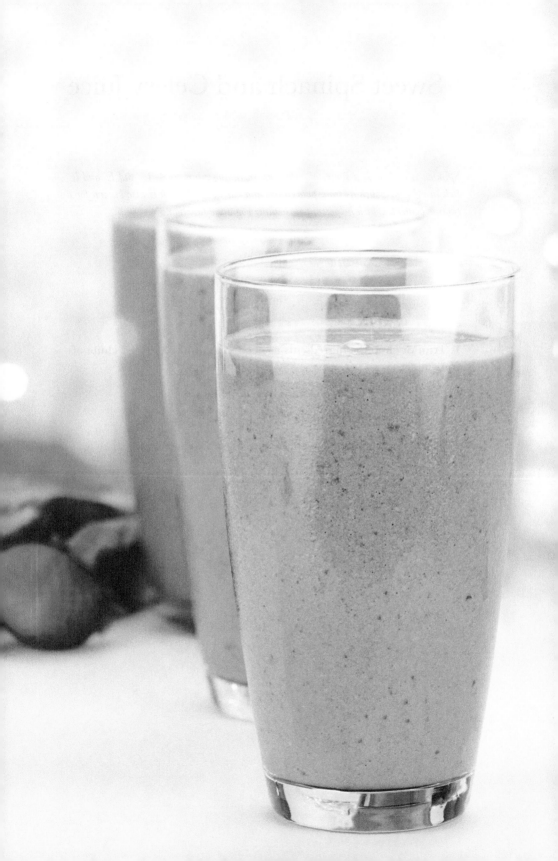

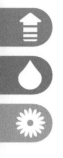

Sweet Spinach and Celery Juice

MAKES 2 TO 3 SERVINGS, 8 TO 10 OUNCES EACH

Spinach is an excellent source of vitamins, including vitamins A, C, and E, and is rich in minerals, such as iron, potassium, and calcium. Spinach is also known for its choline content, which helps support healthy cognitive function.

1 BUNCH OR 2 CUPS SPINACH LEAVES
4 LARGE STALKS CELERY, GREENS INCLUDED
2 MEDIUM GREEN APPLES

1. Trim or chop the ingredients as needed to fit into the feed chute of your juicer.

2. Place a pitcher or container under the spout of the juicer.

3. Feed the ingredients through the juicer in the order listed.

4. Stir the juice briefly; then pour it into glasses and serve immediately.

5. Fresh juice may be refrigerated in an airtight container for up to 3 days.

Asparagus Parsley Power Juice

Asparagus is known for its high antioxidant content, which makes it a powerful tool in slowing the appearance of aging and mitigating the risk for cognitive decline. Asparagus is also a good source of fiber and several key vitamins, including vitamins A, C, E, and K.

1 BUNCH OR 20 ASPARAGUS SPEARS, ENDS TRIMMED
2 LARGE STALKS CELERY, GREENS INCLUDED
½ BUNCH FRESH PARSLEY

1. Trim or chop the ingredients as needed to fit into the feed chute of your juicer.

2. Place a pitcher or container under the spout of the juicer.

3. Feed the ingredients through the juicer in the order listed.

4. Stir the juice briefly; then pour it into glasses and serve immediately.

5. Fresh juice may be refrigerated in an airtight container for up to 3 days.

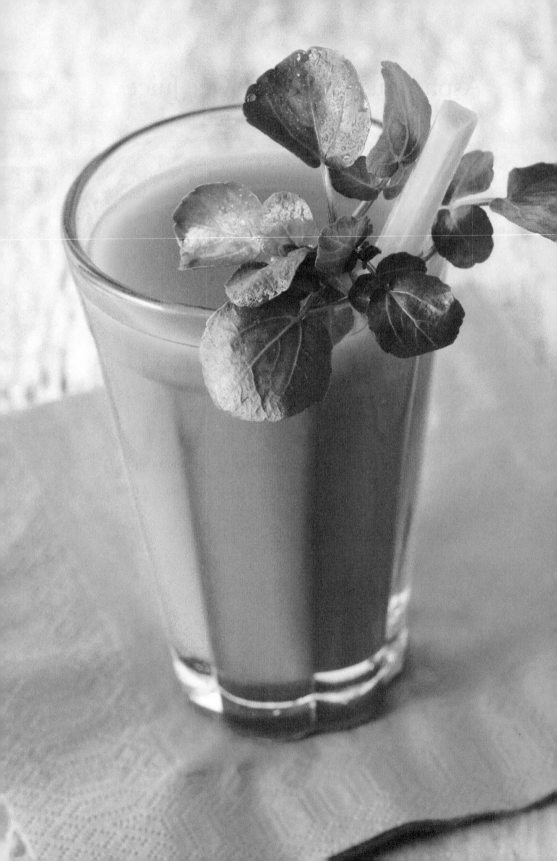

Cleansing Cauliflower Carrot Juice

MAKES 2 TO 3 SERVINGS, 8 TO 10 OUNCES EACH

Cauliflower is rich in a variety of vitamins and minerals, and it also contains glucosinolates, which help support the liver's detoxification abilities, thus cleansing your body of toxins.

1 SMALL HEAD CAULIFLOWER
6 MEDIUM CARROTS
2 LARGE STALKS CELERY
1 LARGE LEAF CURLY KALE
1 GARLIC CLOVE, PEELED
½ LEMON, PEELED

1. Trim or chop the ingredients as needed to fit into the feed chute of your juicer.

2. Place a pitcher or container under the spout of the juicer.

3. Feed the ingredients through the juicer in the order listed.

4. Stir the juice briefly; then pour it into glasses and serve immediately.

5. Fresh juice may be refrigerated in an airtight container for up to 3 days.

Beauty-Boosting Brussels Sprouts Juice

Brussels sprouts are an excellent source of dietary fiber, folate, and potassium. They've also been shown to help improve skin and nail health, which, combined with the sugar snap peas, peach, and orange, makes this recipe both delicious and beauty-boosting!

10 BRUSSELS SPROUTS, TRIMMED
1 CUP SUGAR SNAP PEAS
1 MEDIUM PEACH, PITTED
1 SMALL ORANGE, HALVED AND PEELED

1. Trim or chop the ingredients as needed to fit into the feed chute of your juicer.

2. Place a pitcher or container under the spout of the juicer.

3. Feed the ingredients through the juicer in the order listed.

4. Stir the juice briefly; then pour it into glasses and serve immediately.

5. Fresh juice may be refrigerated in an airtight container for up to 3 days.

Skin-Clearing Celery Juice

MAKES 2 SERVINGS, 8 TO 10 OUNCES EACH

Despite being low in calories, celery is rich in nutrients. It contains multiple types of anti-cancer compounds, including coumarins, which have been shown to repair cellular damage caused by free radicals.

4 LARGE STALKS CELERY

2 ASPARAGUS SPEARS, ENDS TRIMMED

1 SMALL SWEET POTATO

1 SMALL PLUM TOMATO

1 TABLESPOON GROUND FLAXSEED

1. Trim or chop the ingredients as needed to fit into the feed chute of your juicer.

2. Place a pitcher or container under the spout of the juicer.

3. Feed the first 4 ingredients through the juicer in the order listed.

4. Stir the flaxseed into the juice; then pour the juice into glasses and serve immediately.

5. Fresh juice may be refrigerated in an airtight container for up to 3 days.

Ginger Vegetable Juice Blend

Ginger is a root vegetable often used in fresh or dried form as a spice. Raw ginger is known for its detoxification properties, helping cleanse your body and improve digestion.

2 CUPS BABY SPINACH
4 ASPARAGUS SPEARS, ENDS TRIMMED
2 LARGE STALKS CELERY, GREENS INCLUDED
1 LARGE APPLE
½ SEEDLESS CUCUMBER
1 INCH GINGERROOT

1. Trim or chop the ingredients as needed to fit into the feed chute of your juicer.

2. Place a pitcher or container under the spout of the juicer.

3. Feed the ingredients through the juicer in the order listed.

4. Stir the juice briefly; then pour it into glasses and serve immediately.

5. Fresh juice may be refrigerated in an airtight container for up to 3 days.

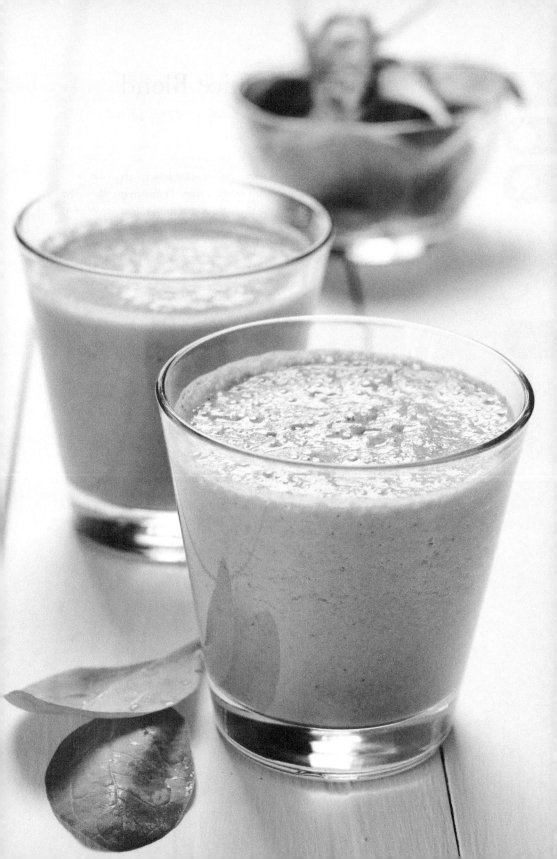

Berry Beet Juice Blend

Beets have been shown to help enhance exercise performance because they contain nutrients that oxygenate the blood, improving recovery time. In this recipe, the oxygen-boosting power of beets combines with the sweet flavor and antioxidant power of fresh blackberries.

6 MEDIUM BEETS, INCLUDING GREENS
1 CUP BLACKBERRIES
1 LARGE CARROT
1 MEDIUM PEAR

1. Trim or chop the ingredients as needed to fit into the feed chute of your juicer.

2. Place a pitcher or container under the spout of the juicer.

3. Feed the ingredients through the juicer in the order listed.

4. Stir the juice briefly; then pour it into glasses and serve immediately.

5. Fresh juice may be refrigerated in an airtight container for up to 3 days.

Antiaging Juice Booster

All of the ingredients in this recipe are known for their antiaging power. Not only will you receive their skin-firming and complexion-enhancing benefits, you'll also get a wide variety of healthful nutrients.

2 MEDIUM PLUM TOMATOES
2 LARGE LEAVES CURLY KALE
1 SMALL RED BELL PEPPER
1 CUP BLACKBERRIES
5 TO 6 FRESH BASIL LEAVES

1. Trim or chop the ingredients as needed to fit into the feed chute of your juicer.

2. Place a pitcher or container under the spout of the juicer.

3. Feed the ingredients through the juicer in the order listed.

4. Stir the juice briefly; then pour it into glasses and serve immediately.

5. Fresh juice may be refrigerated in an airtight container for up to 3 days.

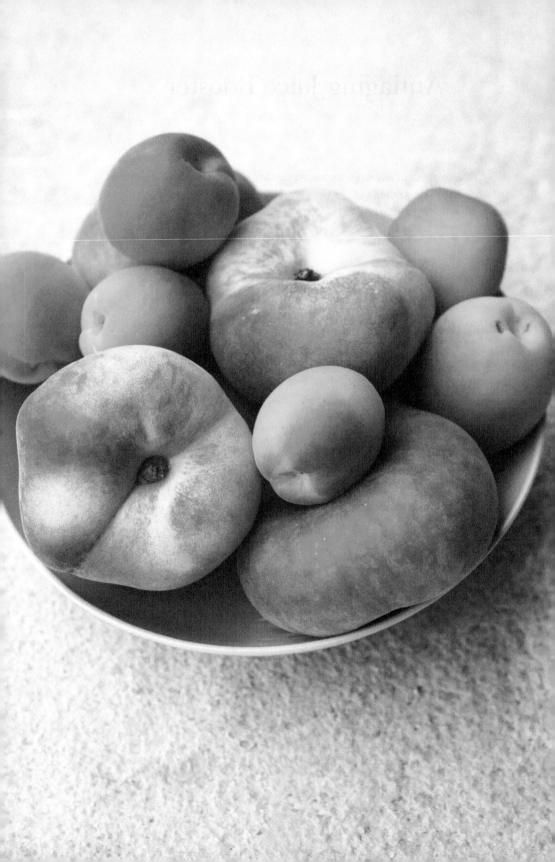

Peachy Parsley Juice

Parsley is known for its healing properties and for its use as a fresh garnish. It contains elements like myristicin that help inhibit tumor growth and promote good overall health.

2 MEDIUM PEACHES, PITTED
1 BUNCH FRESH PARSLEY
½ SMALL HEAD ROMAINE LETTUCE
1 LARGE STALK CELERY

1. Trim or chop the ingredients as needed to fit into the feed chute of your juicer.

2. Place a pitcher or container under the spout of the juicer.

3. Feed the ingredients through the juicer in the order listed.

4. Stir the juice briefly; then pour it into glasses and serve immediately.

5. Fresh juice may be refrigerated in an airtight container for up to 3 days.

Lovely Lime Cilantro Blend

Cilantro and lime are both known for their cool, refreshing flavors. You may not know, however, that cilantro is also rich in antioxidants, making it useful as a digestive aid and an antibacterial agent.

1 BUNCH FRESH CILANTRO

2 LARGE STALKS CELERY

1 LIME, HALVED AND PEELED

1. Trim or chop the ingredients as needed to fit into the feed chute of your juicer.

2. Place a pitcher or container under the spout of the juicer.

3. Feed the ingredients through the juicer in the order listed.

4. Stir the juice briefly; then pour it into glasses and serve immediately.

5. Fresh juice may be refrigerated in an airtight container for up to 3 days.

Just Plain Green Juice

Kohlrabi is a member of the cabbage family and is known for its high vitamin C content—just one cup of kohlrabi contains almost your entire daily dosage. It also contains glucosinolates, which can help protect your body against cancer.

2 MEDIUM KOHLRABI BULBS, GREENS INCLUDED
1 CUP CAULIFLOWER FLORETS
1 SMALL ZUCCHINI
2 TO 3 SPRIGS FRESH THYME

1. Trim or chop the ingredients as needed to fit into the feed chute of your juicer.

2. Place a pitcher or container under the spout of the juicer.

3. Feed the ingredients through the juicer in the order listed.

4. Stir the juice briefly; then pour it into glasses and serve immediately.

5. Fresh juice may be refrigerated in an airtight container for up to 3 days.

Berry Basil Blusher

MAKES 2 SERVINGS, 8 TO 10 OUNCES EACH

Unlike many herbs, basil juices very well in its fresh form. Not only is it full of delicious juice, but its appealing aroma is guaranteed to make any juice more appetizing.

1 SMALL SEEDLESS CUCUMBER
1 CUP CHERRY TOMATOES
½ CUP FRESH BASIL LEAVES, PLUS EXTRA
FOR GARNISH (OPTIONAL)
½ CUP BERRIES (YOUR CHOICE)

1. Trim or chop the ingredients as needed to fit into the feed chute of your juicer.

2. Place a pitcher or container under the spout of the juicer.

3. Feed the ingredients through the juicer in the order listed.

4. Stir the juice briefly; then pour it into glasses and serve immediately.

5. Chop a few extra basil leaves and stir them into the juice for garnish (if using).

6. Fresh juice may be refrigerated in an airtight container for up to 3 days.

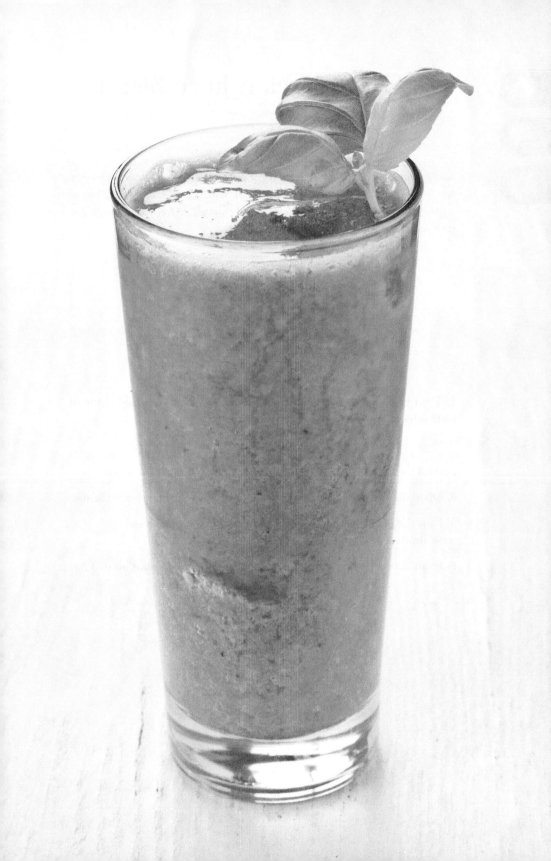

Green Dream Juice Blend

Studies have shown that consuming dark green vegetables and legumes may help calm your nervous system and improve the quality of your sleep. Adding a St. John's wort supplement to a glass of fresh vegetable juice before bed may also help you get the sleep you need.

1 LARGE LEAF SWISS CHARD
1 HANDFUL SUGAR SNAP PEAS
1 STALK CELERY
1 (300 MG) ST. JOHN'S WORT HERBAL SUPPLEMENT CAPSULE
PINCH OF GROUND NUTMEG

1. Trim or chop the ingredients as needed to fit into the feed chute of your juicer.

2. Place a pitcher or container under the spout of the juicer.

3. Feed the first 3 ingredients through the juicer in the order listed.

4. Open the capsule of St. John's wort, and stir the contents into the juice.

5. Pour the juice into a glass; then sprinkle it with nutmeg and serve immediately.

6. Fresh juice may be refrigerated in an airtight container for up to 3 days.

Sweet Swiss Chard Juice

Some of the vegetables with the sweetest natural flavor include sugar snap peas, carrots, and rutabaga. Combined with the nutrient-packed power of Swiss chard, that makes this juice as delicious as it is healthful.

1 BUNCH OR 2 CUPS SWISS CHARD
1 CUP SUGAR SNAP PEAS
1 LARGE CARROT
1 SMALL RUTABAGA
¼ CUP FRESH BASIL LEAVES, PACKED

1. Trim or chop the ingredients as needed to fit into the feed chute of your juicer.

2. Place a pitcher or container under the spout of the juicer.

3. Feed the ingredients through the juicer in the order listed.

4. Stir the juice briefly; then pour it into glasses and serve immediately.

5. Fresh juice may be refrigerated in an airtight container for up to 3 days.

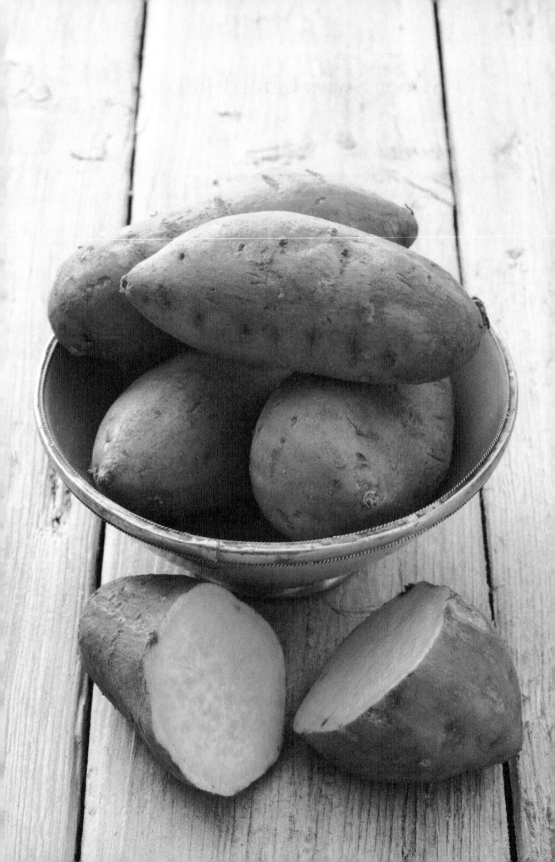

Sweet Potato Protein Spritzer

This recipe packs a powerful punch, full of the protein you need to get you through your day. Not only is it full of vital nutrients, but it also has the delicious flavor of sweet potatoes and apple.

2 MEDIUM SWEET POTATOES
2 CUPS BABY SPINACH LEAVES
1 CUP CHOPPED TURNIP GREENS
1 LARGE CARROT
1 MEDIUM APPLE

1. Trim or chop the ingredients as needed to fit into the feed chute of your juicer.

2. Place a pitcher or container under the spout of the juicer.

3. Feed the ingredients through the juicer in the order listed.

4. Stir the juice briefly; then pour it into glasses and serve immediately.

5. Fresh juice may be refrigerated in an airtight container for up to 3 days.

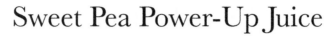

Sweet Pea Power-Up Juice

MAKES 2 TO 3 SERVINGS, 8 TO 10 OUNCES EACH

Pea shoots are sometimes referred to as a microgreen because they are harvested when they are just a few weeks old. These sprouts are loaded with antioxidants as well as folate and carotene, all of which help prevent cancer and repair cellular damage caused by free radicals.

2 SEEDLESS CUCUMBERS
1 CUP SWEET PEA SHOOTS
1 CUP CHOPPED KALE LEAVES
4 STALKS CELERY, INCLUDING GREENS
1 LARGE APPLE
1 INCH GINGERROOT

1. Trim or chop the ingredients as needed to fit into the feed chute of your juicer.

2. Place a pitcher or container under the spout of the juicer.

3. Feed the ingredients through the juicer in the order listed.

4. Stir the juice briefly; then pour it into glasses and serve immediately.

5. Fresh juice may be refrigerated in an airtight container for up to 3 days.

Tasty Tomato Turnip Juice

Turnips belong to the same family as broccoli and kale, making them a cruciferous vegetable. These vegetables provide a wealth of health benefits, but the most significant is their cancer-preventing properties.

2 LARGE PLUM TOMATOES
1 LARGE TURNIP, GREENS INCLUDED
1 LARGE CARROT
3 TO 4 SPRIGS FRESH PARSLEY
PINCH OF DRIED TARRAGON

1. Trim or chop the ingredients as needed to fit into the feed chute of your juicer.

2. Place a pitcher or container under the spout of the juicer.

3. Feed the first 4 ingredients through the juicer in the order listed.

4. Stir the dried tarragon into the juice, then pour the juice into glasses and serve immediately.

5. Fresh juice may be refrigerated in an airtight container for up to 3 days.

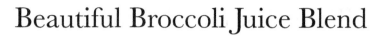

Beautiful Broccoli Juice Blend

MAKES 2 TO 3 SERVINGS, 8 TO 10 OUNCES EACH

Broccoli is a cruciferous vegetable, which means that it is incredibly rich in dietary fiber. This wonderful vegetable also contains high levels of vitamin C, which helps promote healing as well as gum and teeth health.

1 SMALL HEAD BROCCOLI
2 CUPS DANDELION GREENS
1 SMALL GREEN BELL PEPPER
½ LEMON, PEELED
½ BUNCH FRESH CILANTRO LEAVES
2 GARLIC CLOVES, PEELED

1. Trim or chop the ingredients as needed to fit into the feed chute of your juicer.

2. Place a pitcher or container under the spout of the juicer.

3. Feed the ingredients through the juicer in the order listed.

4. Stir the juice briefly; then pour it into glasses and serve immediately.

5. Fresh juice may be refrigerated in an airtight container for up to 3 days.

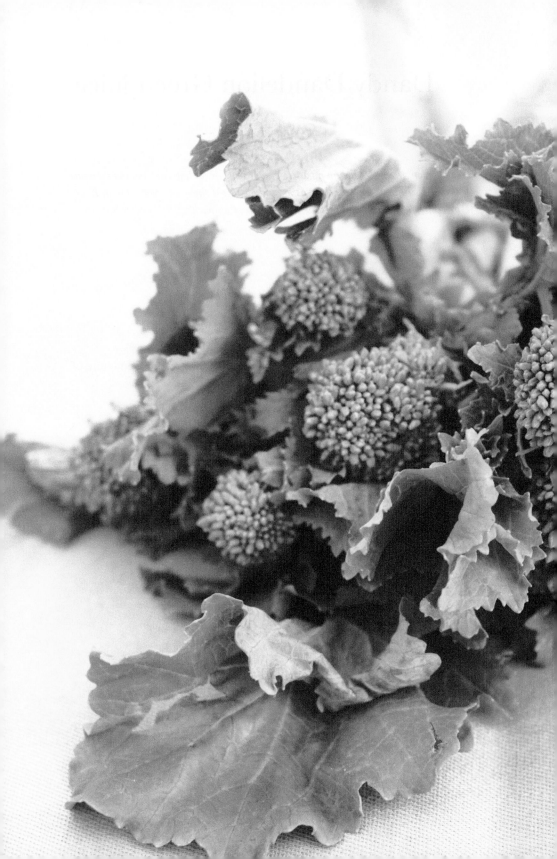

Dandy Dandelion Green Juice

Dandelion greens are rich in a variety of nutrients, including calcium and vitamins C and K. In fact, dandelion greens have almost eight times as much vitamin K as broccoli, as well as two times the iron content of spinach.

3 RADISHES, GREENS INCLUDED
1 BUNCH OR 2 CUPS DANDELION GREENS
1 LARGE LEAF RED CABBAGE
2 PLUMS, PITTED

1. Trim or chop the ingredients as needed to fit into the feed chute of your juicer.

2. Place a pitcher or container under the spout of the juicer.

3. Feed the ingredients through the juicer in the order listed.

4. Stir the juice briefly; then pour it into glasses and serve immediately.

5. Fresh juice may be refrigerated in an airtight container for up to 3 days.

Kale Cabbage Juice

Kale is one of the highest vegetable sources of vitamin K, which is particularly helpful in reducing the risk for certain cancers. It is incredibly nutrient-dense, containing a variety of vitamins and minerals, including iron, phosphorus, calcium, and chlorophyll.

1 BUNCH OR 2 CUPS CURLY KALE
1 LARGE CARROT
½ SMALL HEAD RED CABBAGE
PINCH OF CHINESE FIVE-SPICE POWDER

1. Trim or chop the ingredients as needed to fit into the feed chute of your juicer.

2. Place a pitcher or container under the spout of the juicer.

3. Feed the first 3 ingredients through the juicer in the order listed.

4. Stir the Chinese five-spice powder into the juice; then pour the juice into glasses and serve immediately.

5. Fresh juice may be refrigerated in an airtight container for up to 3 days.

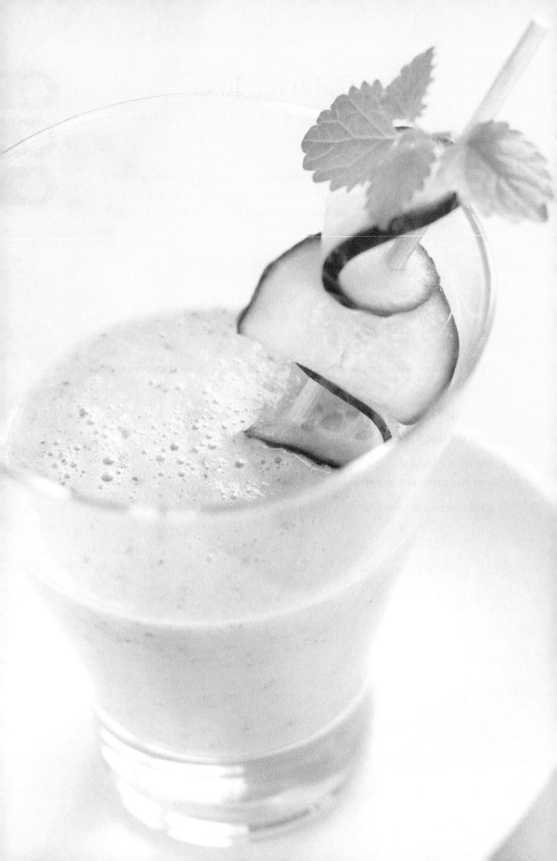

Turnip Celery Juicer

Some of the health benefits associated with turnips include high concentrations of calcium, magnesium, and potassium, as well as vitamins C and K.

4 LARGE STALKS CELERY
2 MEDIUM TURNIPS, GREENS INCLUDED
1 SMALL ENGLISH CUCUMBER
2 TO 3 SPRIGS FRESH MINT, FOR GARNISH

1. Trim or chop the ingredients as needed to fit into the feed chute of your juicer.

2. Place a pitcher or container under the spout of the juicer.

3. Feed the first 3 ingredients through the juicer in the order listed.

4. Stir the juice briefly; then pour it into glasses.

5. Garnish with the sprigs of fresh mint to serve.

6. Fresh juice may be refrigerated in an airtight container for up to 3 days.

Radish Rutabaga Juice Blend

MAKES 2 SERVINGS, 8 TO 10 OUNCES EACH

Rutabaga is sometimes referred to as yellow turnip and is well known for its vitamin C content, which has been shown to reduce the risk for certain cancers.

6 MEDIUM RADISHES, GREENS INCLUDED
1 MEDIUM RUTABAGA
1 SMALL SWEET POTATO
4 TO 6 FRESH BASIL LEAVES

1. Trim or chop the ingredients as needed to fit into the feed chute of your juicer.

2. Place a pitcher or container under the spout of the juicer.

3. Feed the ingredients through the juicer in the order listed.

4. Stir the juice briefly; then pour it into glasses and serve immediately.

5. Fresh juice may be refrigerated in an airtight container for up to 3 days.

Brilliant Brussels Sprouts Juice

Brussels sprouts are an excellent vegetable if you're trying to lower or control your cholesterol levels. They have a high fiber content and a variety of enzymes that help to keep your heart healthy.

8 BRUSSELS SPROUTS, TRIMMED
1 CUP CAULIFLOWER FLORETS
1 SMALL BULB CELERIAC
3 TO 5 DROPS ALOE VERA JUICE

1. Trim or chop the ingredients as needed to fit into the feed chute of your juicer.

2. Place a pitcher or container under the spout of the juicer.

3. Feed the first 3 ingredients through the juicer in the order listed.

4. Stir aloe vera juice into the juice; then pour the juice into glasses and serve immediately.

5. Fresh juice may be refrigerated in an airtight container for up to 3 days.

Blueberry Beetroot Booster

Beets have been linked to a variety of health benefits, including improved stamina and blood flow as well as decreased blood pressure.

6 MEDIUM BEETS, GREENS INCLUDED
2 LARGE CARROTS
1 LARGE STALK CELERY
1 CUP BLUEBERRIES
2 SPRIGS FRESH PARSLEY, FOR GARNISH

1. Trim or chop the ingredients as needed to fit into the feed chute of your juicer.

2. Place a pitcher or container under the spout of the juicer.

3. Feed the first 4 ingredients through the juicer in the order listed.

4. Stir the juice briefly; then pour it into glasses.

5. Garnish with the sprigs of fresh parsley to serve.

6. Fresh juice may be refrigerated in an airtight container for up to 3 days.

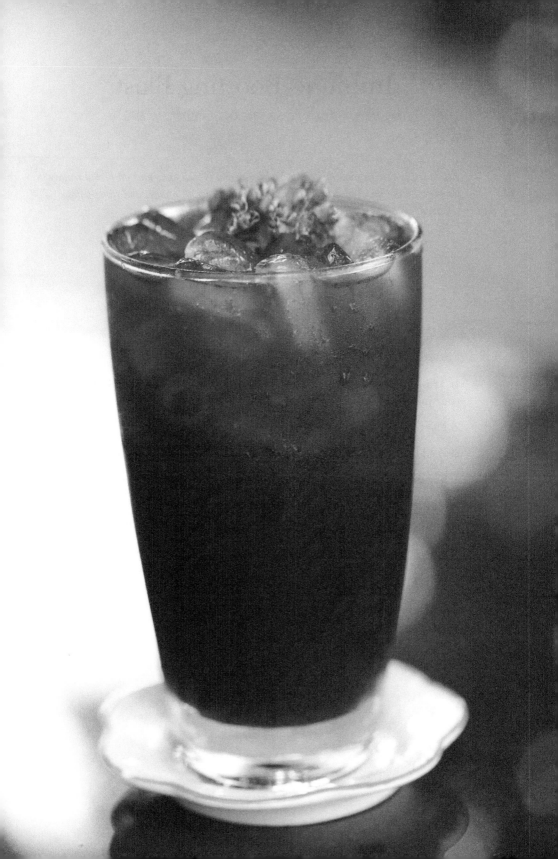

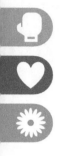

Immune-Boosting Blast

MAKES 2 SERVINGS, 8 TO 10 OUNCES EACH

Echinacea is derived from the purple coneflower and is well known as an herbal remedy for the cold and flu. Added to fresh juice made with carrots, orange, and sweet potato, echinacea improves the immune-boosting power of this recipe.

2 LARGE CARROTS
1 MEDIUM ORANGE, HALVED AND PEELED
1 MEDIUM SWEET POTATO
1 SMALL MANGO, PITTED
1 TEASPOON ECHINACEA

1. Trim or chop the ingredients as needed to fit into the feed chute of your juicer.

2. Place a pitcher or container under the spout of the juicer.

3. Feed the first 4 ingredients through the juicer in the order listed.

4. Stir the echinacea into the juice; then pour the juice into glasses and serve immediately.

5. Fresh juice may be refrigerated in an airtight container for up to 3 days.

Brain Power Beet Juice Blend

Beets are an excellent source of natural nitrates, which can help increase blood flow to the brain, thus improving your cognitive performance.

6 MEDIUM BEETS, GREENS INCLUDED
2 CUPS CHOPPED MUSTARD GREENS
1 SMALL SUMMER SQUASH

1. Trim or chop the ingredients as needed to fit into the feed chute of your juicer.

2. Place a pitcher or container under the spout of the juicer.

3. Feed the ingredients through the juicer in the order listed.

4. Stir the juice briefly; then pour it into glasses and serve immediately.

5. Fresh juice may be refrigerated in an airtight container for up to 3 days.

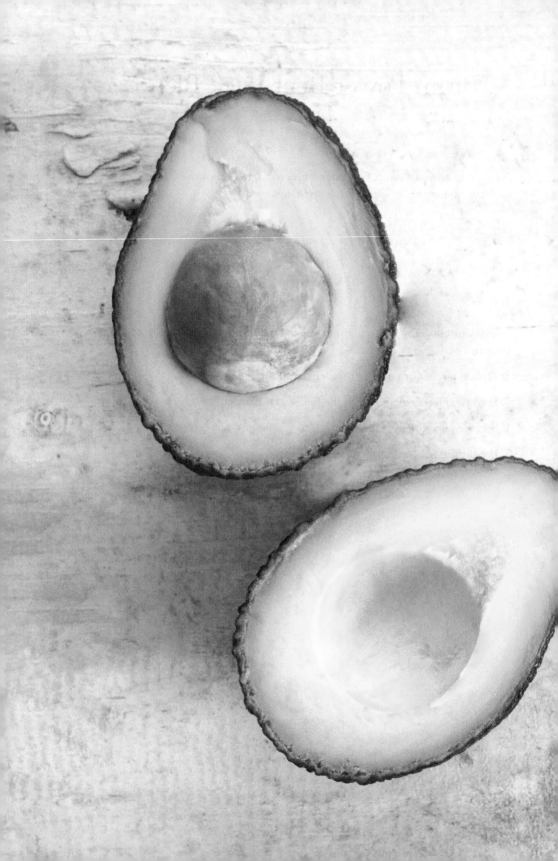

Avocado Asparagus Juice

MAKES 2 TO 3 SERVINGS, 8 TO 10 OUNCES EACH

Due to its soft texture, avocado cannot be passed through your juicer. To include it in this recipe you'll need to juice the other ingredients and then blend the juice with the avocado in a blender.

½ BUNCH OR 10 ASPARAGUS SPEARS, ENDS TRIMMED
2 LARGE STALKS CELERY
½ MEDIUM SEEDLESS CUCUMBER
1 CUP FRESH CILANTRO LEAVES, PACKED
1 AVOCADO, PEELED AND PITTED

1. Trim or chop the ingredients as needed to fit into the feed chute of your juicer.

2. Place a pitcher or container under the spout of the juicer.

3. Feed the first 4 ingredients through the juicer in the order listed.

4. Stir the juice briefly; then pour it into a blender.

5. Add the avocado and blend until smooth.

6. Pour the mixture into glasses to serve.

7. Fresh juice may be refrigerated in an airtight container for up to 3 days; wait until you're ready to consume the juice to add the avocado.

Spinach Cucumber Celery Juice

Spinach, cucumber, and celery are all excellent vegetables for juicing due to their high water content and concentration of nutrients. This juice recipe is full of flavor and healthful benefits—not to mention the fact that it's incredibly refreshing.

1 HOTHOUSE CUCUMBER
1 BUNCH OR 2 CUPS SPINACH LEAVES
2 LARGE STALKS CELERY
½ LIME, PEELED

1. Trim or chop the ingredients as needed to fit into the feed chute of your juicer.

2. Place a pitcher or container under the spout of the juicer.

3. Feed the ingredients through the juicer in the order listed.

4. Stir the juice briefly; then pour it into glasses and serve immediately.

5. Fresh juice may be refrigerated in an airtight container for up to 3 days.

Protein-Packed Juice Blend

You don't have to eat a big piece of chicken or steak to meet your daily requirements for protein. Many vegetables, including kale, broccoli, and collard greens, are a good source of vegetarian protein.

1 BUNCH OR 2 CUPS CURLY KALE
1 SMALL HEAD BROCCOLI
½ BUNCH OR 1 CUP COLLARD GREENS
1 LARGE CARROT
2 TABLESPOONS GROUND FLAXSEED

1. Trim or chop the ingredients as needed to fit into the feed chute of your juicer.

2. Place a pitcher or container under the spout of the juicer.

3. Feed the first 4 ingredients through the juicer in the order listed.

4. Stir the flaxseed into the juice; then pour the juice into glasses and serve immediately.

5. Fresh juice may be refrigerated in an airtight container for up to 3 days.

Fennel Apple Juice Booster

This recipe combines the crisp, refreshing flavor of fennel with the lightly sweet flavor of ripe apples.

2 LARGE APPLES
2 LARGE STALKS CELERY
1 MEDIUM FENNEL BULB
¼ SMALL HEAD GREEN CABBAGE

1. Trim or chop the ingredients as needed to fit into the feed chute of your juicer.

2. Place a pitcher or container under the spout of the juicer.

3. Feed the ingredients through the juicer in the order listed.

4. Stir the juice briefly; then pour it into a glass and serve immediately.

5. Fresh juice may be refrigerated in an airtight container for up to 3 days.

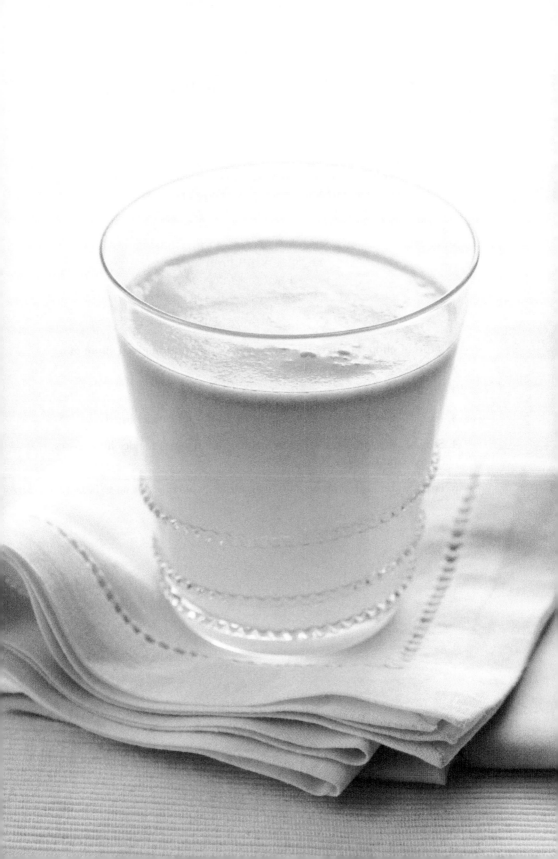

Green Machine Juice Blend

The ingredients in this recipe are packed with healthful nutrients shown to boost energy levels, giving you exactly what you need to power through your day.

1 BUNCH OR 2 CUPS COLLARD GREENS
1 MEDIUM KOHLRABI BULB
1 CUP BROCCOLI FLORETS
1 TABLESPOON WHEATGRASS POWDER

1. Trim or chop the ingredients as needed to fit into the feed chute of your juicer.

2. Place a pitcher or container under the spout of the juicer.

3. Feed the first 3 ingredients through the juicer in the order listed.

4. Stir the wheatgrass powder into the juice; then pour the juice into glasses and serve immediately.

5. Fresh juice may be refrigerated in an airtight container for up to 3 days.

Wrinkle-Reducing Cucumber Juice

MAKES 2 TO 3 SERVINGS, 8 TO 10 OUNCES EACH

Studies have shown that increasing your intake of unsaturated fats may help reduce wrinkles by improving your skin's defense against sun damage. Here, leafy green vegetables like spinach and bok choy help boost these defenses, while cucumber juice adds cool, refreshing flavor.

1 HOTHOUSE CUCUMBER
1 BUNCH OR 2 CUPS SPINACH LEAVES
1 CUP CHOPPED BOK CHOY
½ LIME, PEELED

1. Trim or chop the ingredients as needed to fit into the feed chute of your juicer.

2. Place a pitcher or container under the spout of the juicer.

3. Feed the ingredients through the juicer in the order listed.

4. Stir the juice briefly; then pour it into glasses and serve immediately.

5. Fresh juice may be refrigerated in an airtight container for up to 3 days.

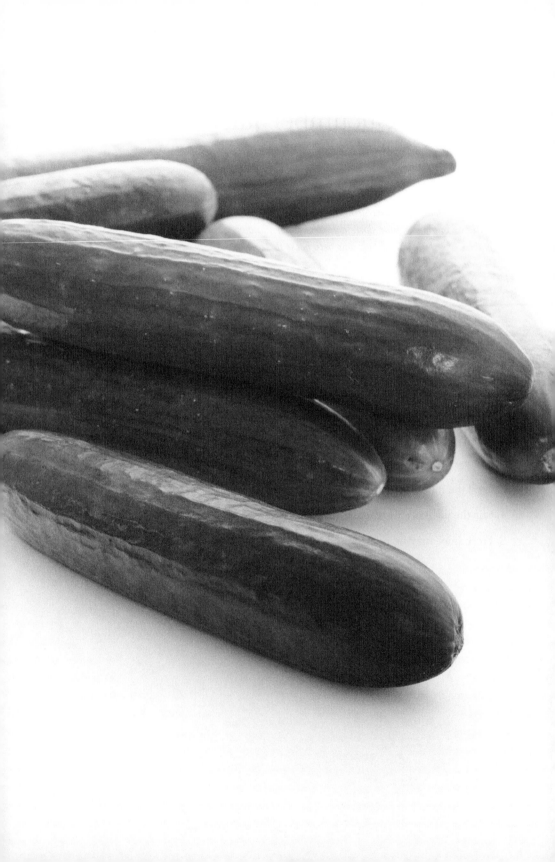

Green Carrot Broccoli Juice

Broccoli is one of those dark green vegetables known for a high nutrient content. In this recipe you also get the detoxifying benefit of carrots and cucumber to top things off.

1 MEDIUM HEAD BROCCOLI
2 LARGE CARROTS
1 SMALL SEEDLESS CUCUMBER
1 MEDIUM APPLE
3 SPRIGS FRESH MINT, FOR GARNISH

1. Trim or chop the ingredients as needed to fit into the feed chute of your juicer.

2. Place a pitcher or container under the spout of the juicer.

3. Feed the first 4 ingredients through the juicer in the order listed.

4. Stir the juice briefly; then pour it into glasses and garnish with fresh mint to serve.

5. Fresh juice may be refrigerated in an airtight container for up to 3 days.

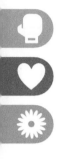

Wonderful Weight-Loss Juice

One of the secrets to weight loss is increasing your water intake. Fruits and vegetables like watermelon, celery, and romaine lettuce are known for their water content, which makes them an excellent addition to this recipe.

1 SMALL BUNCH OR 2 CUPS ROMAINE LETTUCE
2 LARGE STALKS CELERY
1 CUP CHOPPED SEEDLESS WATERMELON, RIND REMOVED
3 TO 4 SPRIGS FRESH CILANTRO OR PARSLEY

1. Trim or chop the ingredients as needed to fit into the feed chute of your juicer.

2. Place a pitcher or container under the spout of the juicer.

3. Feed the ingredients through the juicer in the order listed.

4. Stir the juice briefly; then pour it into glasses and serve immediately.

5. Fresh juice may be refrigerated in an airtight container for up to 3 days.

Hearty Beet and
Dandelion Green Juice

This hearty juice is packed with flavor and healthful nutrients. Enjoy it as an afternoon snack or a nutritious breakfast beverage.

1 BUNCH OR 2 CUPS DANDELION GREENS
4 MEDIUM BEETS, GREENS INCLUDED
2 MEDIUM SCALLIONS
1 LARGE CARROT

1. Trim or chop the ingredients as needed to fit into the feed chute of your juicer.

2. Place a pitcher or container under the spout of the juicer.

3. Feed the ingredients through the juicer in the order listed.

4. Stir the juice briefly; then pour it into glasses and serve immediately.

5. Fresh juice may be refrigerated in an airtight container for up to 3 days.

Awesome Arugula Tonic

When fresh, arugula has an attractive dark green color. Don't use it if the leaves have turned yellow, because this means it is no longer fresh.

1 LARGE BUNCH OR 2 CUPS FRESH ARUGULA
2 LARGE STALKS CELERY
1 LARGE CARROT
1 SMALL TURNIP, GREENS INCLUDED

1. Trim or chop the ingredients as needed to fit into the feed chute of your juicer.

2. Place a pitcher or container under the spout of the juicer.

3. Feed the ingredients through the juicer in the order listed.

4. Stir the juice briefly; then pour it into glasses and serve immediately.

5. Fresh juice may be refrigerated in an container for up to 3 days.

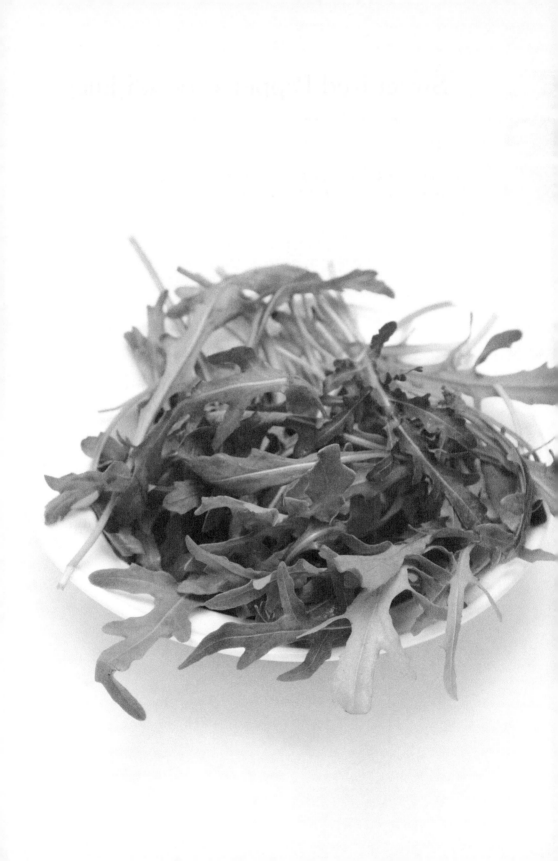

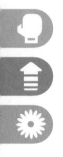

Sweet Red Pepper Broccoli Juice

MAKES 2 TO 3 SERVINGS, 8 TO 10 OUNCES EACH

Bell peppers are known for their high levels of vitamin C, a vitamin that is essential for eye and gum health. It also helps promote healing.

2 LARGE LEAVES CURLY KALE
1 CUP BABY SPINACH LEAVES, PACKED
1 CUP BROCCOLI FLORETS
1 LARGE RED BELL PEPPER
1 LARGE PEAR
¼ TEASPOON GROUND CUMIN

1. Trim or chop the ingredients as needed to fit into the feed chute of your juicer.

2. Place a pitcher or container under the spout of the juicer.

3. Feed the first 5 ingredients through the juicer in the order listed.

4. Stir the cumin into the juice; then pour the juice into glasses and serve immediately.

5. Fresh juice may be refrigerated in an airtight container for up to 3 days.

Tasty Turnip Green Juice

Sage has a lightly sweet flavor that pairs well with the fresh turnip greens and ripe tomatoes in this recipe. Add to that its rich vitamin K content, and this juice is bursting with healthful nutrients.

1 BUNCH OR 2 CUPS TURNIP GREENS
2 SMALL RADISHES, GREENS INCLUDED
1 MEDIUM PLUM TOMATO
2 SPRIGS FRESH SAGE

1. Trim or chop the ingredients as needed to fit into the feed chute of your juicer.

2. Place a pitcher or container under the spout of the juicer.

3. Feed the ingredients through the juicer in the order listed.

4. Stir the juice briefly; then pour it into glasses and serve immediately.

5. Fresh juice may be refrigerated in an airtight container for up to 3 days.

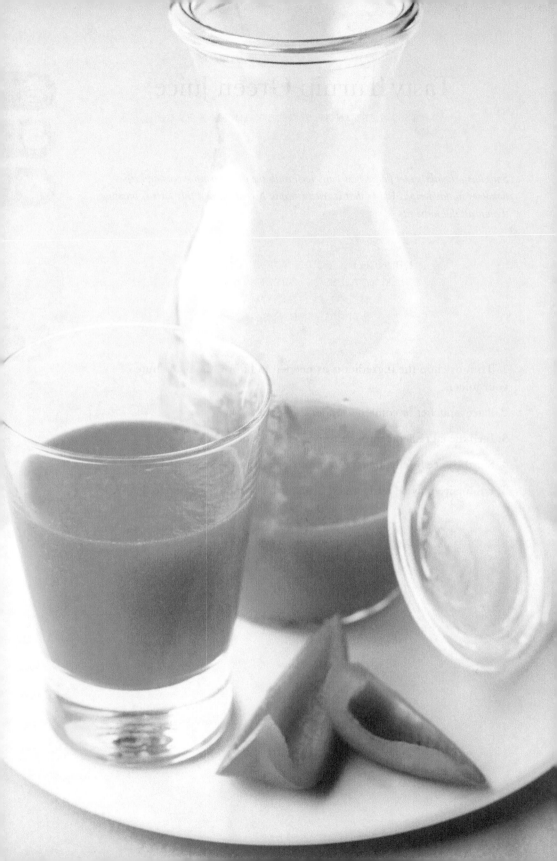

Rockin' Red Pepper Juice

Bell peppers come in a variety of different colors, and all of them are rich in vitamins A and C. Vitamin C helps promote healing, while vitamin A is essential for maintaining skin and eye health.

2 RED BELL PEPPERS
2 MEDIUM TART RED APPLES
1 LARGE CARROT
1 LARGE STALK CELERY, GREENS INCLUDED
½ CUP STRAWBERRIES

1. Trim or chop the ingredients as needed to fit into the feed chute of your juicer.

2. Place a pitcher or container under the spout of the juicer.

3. Feed the ingredients through the juicer in the order listed.

4. Stir the juice briefly; then pour it into glasses and serve immediately.

5. Fresh juice may be refrigerated in an airtight container for up to 3 days.

Cool Celery Limeade

If you're looking for a healthful beverage to help you cool down on a hot day, this celery limeade is exactly what you've been searching for. Stir in a few mint leaves to make it even more refreshing.

4 LARGE STALKS CELERY
2 LARGE LEAVES ROMAINE LETTUCE
2 LIMES, HALVED AND PEELED
HANDFUL FRESH MINT LEAVES

1. Trim or chop the ingredients as needed to fit into the feed chute of your juicer.

2. Place a pitcher or container under the spout of the juicer.

3. Feed the first 3 ingredients through the juicer in the order listed.

4. Stir the mint leaves into the juice; then pour the juice into glasses and serve immediately.

5. Fresh juice may be refrigerated in an airtight container for up to 3 days.

Carrot Orange Ginger Juice

All of the ingredients in this recipe are known for their detox-boosting properties. On top of that, the flavors of carrot, ginger, and orange blend perfectly to create a flavorful, refreshing juice.

4 LARGE CARROTS
2 ORANGES, HALVED AND PEELED
½ SEEDLESS CUCUMBER
½ INCH GINGERROOT

1. Trim or chop the ingredients as needed to fit into the feed chute of your juicer.

2. Place a pitcher or container under the spout of the juicer.

3. Feed the ingredients through the juicer in the order listed.

4. Stir the juice briefly; then pour it into glasses and serve immediately.

5. Fresh juice may be refrigerated in an airtight container for up to 3 days.

Homegrown Green Juice

This recipe is the perfect way to use the vegetables from your backyard garden. Feel free to swap out one or two of the ingredients listed for whatever fresh vegetables you have in season.

2 LARGE LEAVES CURLY KALE
2 LARGE LEAVES ROMAINE LETTUCE
1 LARGE CARROT
1 LARGE STALK CELERY
3 TO 4 SPRIGS FRESH MINT

1. Trim or chop the ingredients as needed to fit into the feed chute of your juicer.

2. Place a pitcher or container under the spout of the juicer.

3. Feed the ingredients through the juicer in the order listed.

4. Stir the juice briefly; then pour it into glasses and serve immediately.

5. Fresh juice may be refrigerated in an airtight container for up to 3 days.

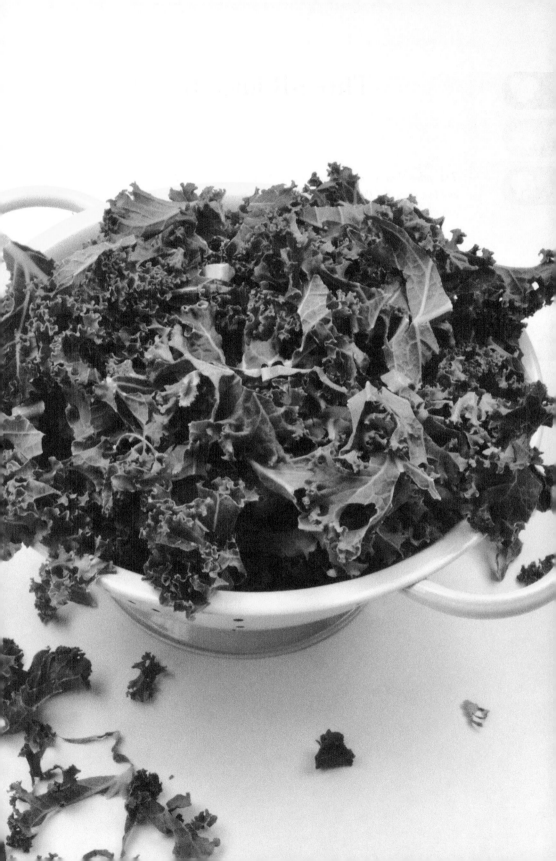

Three-B Juice Blend

This juice blend is made from a triple threat of vegetables: Brussels sprouts, broccoli, and bok choy. All three are rich in dietary fiber and contain a variety of essential vitamins and minerals.

10 BRUSSELS SPROUTS, TRIMMED
2 CUPS BROCCOLI FLORETS
2 CUPS CHOPPED BOK CHOY LEAVES
1 MEDIUM APPLE

1. Trim or chop the ingredients as needed to fit into the feed chute of your juicer.

2. Place a pitcher or container under the spout of the juicer.

3. Feed the ingredients through the juicer in the order listed.

4. Stir the juice briefly; then pour it into glasses and serve immediately.

5. Fresh juice may be refrigerated in an airtight container for up to 3 days.

Green Bean Sprout Power Juice

When it comes to juicing, bean sprouts may not be the first ingredient you think of. These sprouts, however, are rich in vitamins B and C, and they're also one of the few vegetables that continue to increase in nutritional value after being picked.

1 CUP BROCCOLI FLORETS
1 CUP GREEN SEEDLESS GRAPES
1 MEDIUM PEAR
½ CUP BEAN SPROUTS

1. Trim or chop the ingredients as needed to fit into the feed chute of your juicer.

2. Place a pitcher or container under the spout of the juicer.

3. Feed the ingredients through the juicer in the order listed.

4. Stir the juice briefly; then pour it into glasses and serve immediately.

5. Fresh juice may be refrigerated in an airtight container for up to 3 days.

Kickin' Kale Collard Green Juice

MAKES 2 TO 3 SERVINGS, 8 TO 10 OUNCES EACH

Kale is an incredibly versatile vegetable, and it is also the highest vegetable source of vitamin K. In combination with the antioxidant content of collard greens, the kale in this juice provides excellent anti-cancer benefits.

1 BUNCH OR 2 CUPS CURLY KALE
1 BUNCH OR 2 CUPS COLLARD GREENS
2 LARGE STALKS CELERY, GREENS INCLUDED
1 INCH GINGERROOT

1. Trim or chop the ingredients as needed to fit into the feed chute of your juicer.

2. Place a pitcher or container under the spout of the juicer.

3. Feed the ingredients through the juicer in the order listed.

4. Stir the juice briefly; then pour it into glasses and serve immediately.

5. Fresh juice may be refrigerated in an airtight container for up to 3 days.

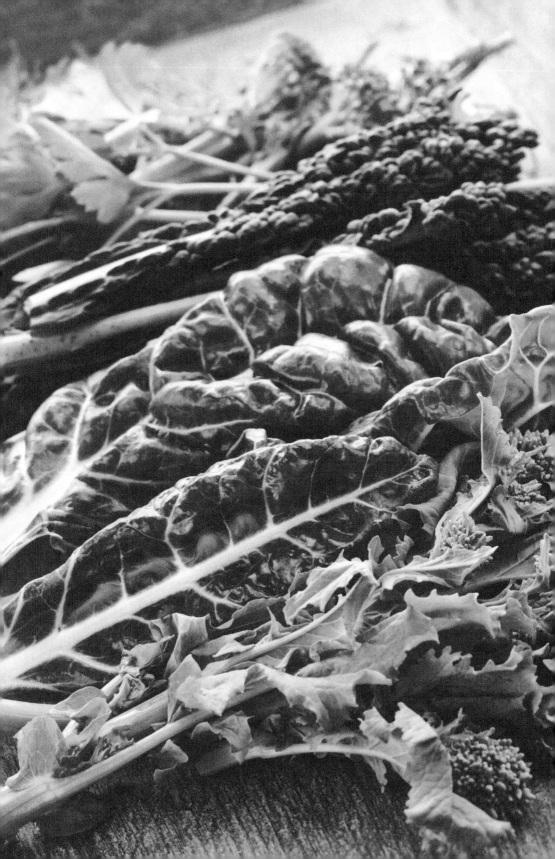

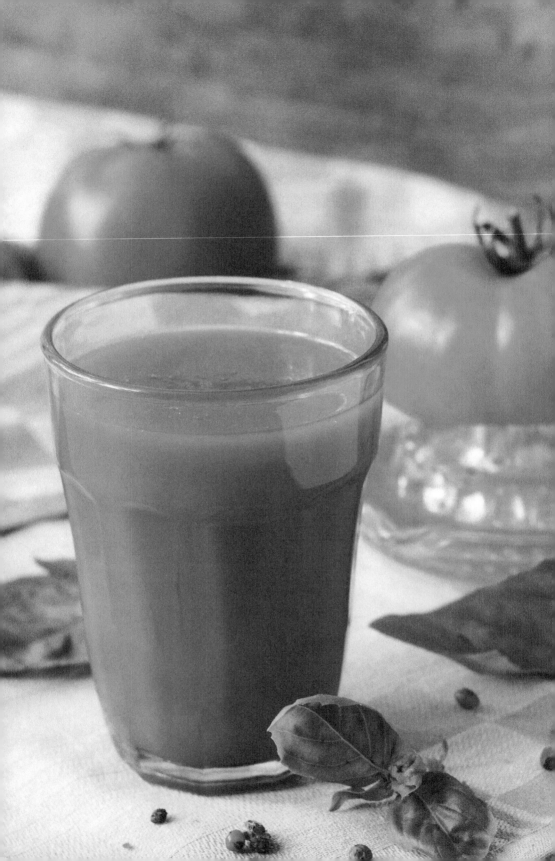

CHAPTER SIXTEEN

30 Savory and Spicy Juices

Curried Juice Cocktail

Sweet Basil Lemonade

Spicy Tomato Juice Blend

Basil Ginger Juice Blend

Garlic Chili Juice Cocktail

Spiced Tropical Island Juice

Cinnamon Pumpkin Juice

Lemon Cayenne Juice Cocktail

Spiced Beet Lemonade

Sweet and Spicy Green Juice

Go-Go Grapefruit Juice

Lean Mean Green Juice Blend

Hot Spiced Nectarine Juice

Indian-Style Green Mango Juice

Spicy Carrot Ginger Juice

Red-Hot V-6 Juice

Raw Spiced Lemonade

Cayenne Red Pepper Juice Blend

Spicy Sunrise Juice Blend

Tart and Tangy Tomato Juice

Spiced Apple Pie Juice

Wasabi Watermelon Juice

Spicy Apple Detox Tonic

Jalapeño Hangover Juice Blend

Pineapple Orange with a Kick

Fiery Fig Mango Juice

Jump-Start Jicama Juice

Raving Red Radish Juice Blend

Spicy Alkaline Juice Mixer

Savory Spring Green Juice

Curried Juice Cocktail

MAKES 3 SERVINGS, 8 TO 10 OUNCES EACH

Curry may not be a flavor you typically associate with juice, but in this juice cocktail, it pulls together the flavors perfectly.

2 CUPS CHOPPED SEEDLESS WATERMELON, RIND REMOVED
2 STALKS CELERY
1 LARGE CARROT
1 ORANGE, HALVED AND PEELED
1½ CUPS COCONUT WATER
1 TEASPOON GROUND CURRY

1. Trim or cut the ingredients as needed to fit into the feed chute of your juicer.

2. Place a pitcher or container under the spout of the juicer.

3. Feed the first 4 ingredients through the juicer in the order listed.

4. Stir the coconut water and ground curry into the juice; then pour the juice into glasses and serve immediately.

5. Fresh juice may be refrigerated in an airtight container for up to 3 days.

Sweet Basil Lemonade

This sweet basil lemonade is a cool and refreshing beverage, the ideal drink to enjoy on a warm evening. If you're looking for a little bit of extra flavor, add a cup of fresh strawberries or raspberries to the mix.

2 LARGE LEMONS, HALVED AND PEELED
½ BUNCH FRESH BASIL LEAVES
2 TABLESPOONS RAW HONEY (OPTIONAL)
COLD WATER TO DILUTE

1. Trim or chop the lemons as needed to fit into the feed chute of your juicer.

2. Place a pitcher or container under the spout of the juicer.

3. Feed the lemons through the juicer and then add the basil.

4. Stir the honey into the juice (if using), and then divide the mixture among 4 glasses.

5. Fill the glasses the rest of the way with cold water, and serve immediately.

6. Fresh juice may be refrigerated in an airtight container for up to 3 days.

Spicy Tomato Juice Blend

Though the juice may still be spicy, the fresh basil in this recipe provides a contrasting, sweeter flavor. If it's still too spicy for you, use only half of the jalapeño pepper.

6 MEDIUM PLUM TOMATOES
2 LARGE STALKS CELERY
1 JALAPEÑO PEPPER, SEEDED
½ BUNCH FRESH BASIL LEAVES

1. Trim or chop the ingredients as needed to fit into the feed chute of your juicer.

2. Place a pitcher or container under the spout of the juicer.

3. Feed the ingredients through the juicer in the order listed.

4. Stir the juice briefly; then pour it into glasses and serve immediately.

5. Fresh juice may be refrigerated in an airtight container for up to 3 days.

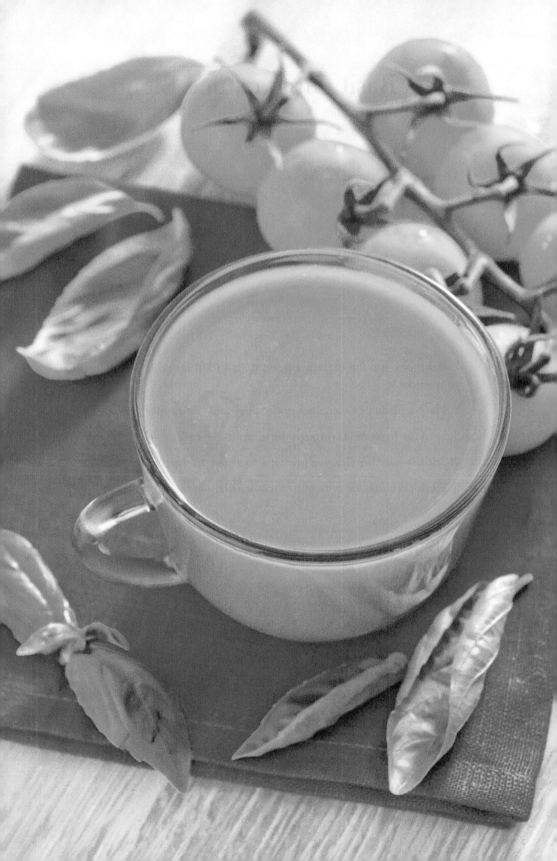

Basil Ginger Juice Blend

This recipe is the ultimate savory juice: the perfect blend of crisp carrots and apples with fresh basil and ginger.

6 LARGE CARROTS
2 MEDIUM APPLES
1 LEMON, HALVED AND PEELED
¼ CUP FRESH BASIL LEAVES, PACKED
1 INCH GINGERROOT

1. Trim or chop the ingredients as needed to fit into the feed chute of your juicer.

2. Place a pitcher or container under the spout of the juicer.

3. Feed the ingredients through the juicer in the order listed.

4. Stir the juice briefly; then pour it into glasses and serve immediately.

5. Fresh juice may be refrigerated in an airtight container for up to 3 days.

Garlic Chili Juice Cocktail

This juice cocktail is a unique and spicy blend of flavors. From tomato and celery to garlic and red chili, your taste buds won't know what to do with themselves.

3 MEDIUM ROMA TOMATOES
2 LARGE STALKS CELERY
1 LARGE CARROT
1 SMALL RED CHILI
1 GARLIC CLOVE, PEELED
PINCH OF CAYENNE PEPPER

1. Trim or chop the ingredients as needed to fit into the feed chute of your juicer.

2. Place a pitcher or container under the spout of the juicer.

3. Feed the first 5 ingredients through the juicer in the order listed.

4. Stir the cayenne pepper into the juice; then pour the juice into glasses and serve immediately.

5. Fresh juice may be refrigerated in an airtight container for up to 3 days.

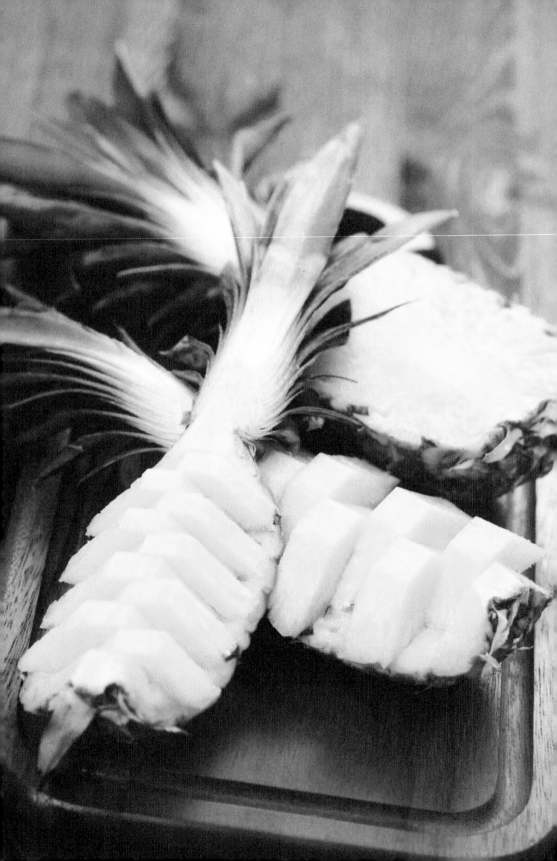

Spiced Tropical Island Juice

Full of fun tropical flavor and a hint of ginger, this spiced tropical island juice will make you feel like you're relaxing in a hammock by the beach.

2 KIWIS, PEELED

2 LARGE STALKS CELERY

1 CUP CHOPPED PINEAPPLE, CORED AND HUSKED

1 MANGO, PEELED AND PITTED

1 MEDIUM APPLE

½ INCH GINGERROOT

1. Trim or chop the ingredients as needed to fit into the feed chute of your juicer.

2. Place a pitcher or container under the spout of the juicer.

3. Feed the ingredients through the juicer in the order listed.

4. Stir the juice briefly; then pour it into glasses and serve immediately.

5. Fresh juice may be refrigerated in an airtight container for up to 3 days.

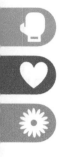

Cinnamon Pumpkin Juice

This cinnamon pumpkin juice is the perfect fall recipe. Feel free to used canned pumpkin puree (not pumpkin pie filling), or make your own from fresh pumpkin.

6 MEDIUM APPLES
1 CUP PUMPKIN PUREE
1 TEASPOON GROUND CINNAMON
PINCH OF GROUND NUTMEG

1. Trim or chop the apples as needed to fit into the feed chute of your juicer.

2. Place a pitcher or container under the spout of the juicer.

3. Feed the apples through the juicer.

4. Stir the pumpkin puree, cinnamon, and nutmeg into the juice.

5. Strain the juice and discard the solids, if desired, before serving.

6. Pour the juice into glasses and serve immediately.

7. Fresh juice may be refrigerated in an airtight container for up to 3 days.

Lemon Cayenne Juice Cocktail

This lemon cayenne juice cocktail was inspired by the infamous "lemonade diet." Though it's not recommended that you live off this juice for several days at a time, it can certainly help detox your body as part of a healthful juice cleanse.

1 MEDIUM LEMON, HALVED AND PEELED
1 TABLESPOON GRADE B MAPLE SYRUP (OPTIONAL)
PINCH OF CAYENNE PEPPER
WATER TO DILUTE

1. Chop the lemons as needed to fit into the feed chute of your juicer.

2. Place a pitcher or container under the spout of the juicer.

3. Feed the lemons through the juicer.

4. Stir the maple syrup (if using) and cayenne into the juice; then pour the juice into glasses.

5. Top the glasses off with water and serve immediately.

6. Fresh juice may be refrigerated in an airtight container for up to 3 days.

Spiced Beet Lemonade

Beet and lemon may sound like a strange combination, but you'll find that it's strangely refreshing.

4 LARGE BEETS, GREENS INCLUDED
3 MEDIUM LEMONS, HALVED AND PEELED
1 CUP WATER
PINCH OF CAYENNE PEPPER

1. Trim or chop the beets and lemons as needed to fit into the feed chute of your juicer.

2. Place a pitcher or container under the spout of the juicer.

3. Feed the beets through the juicer and then the lemons.

4. Stir the water and cayenne pepper into the juice; then pour the juice into glasses and serve immediately.

5. Fresh juice may be refrigerated in an airtight container for up to 3 days.

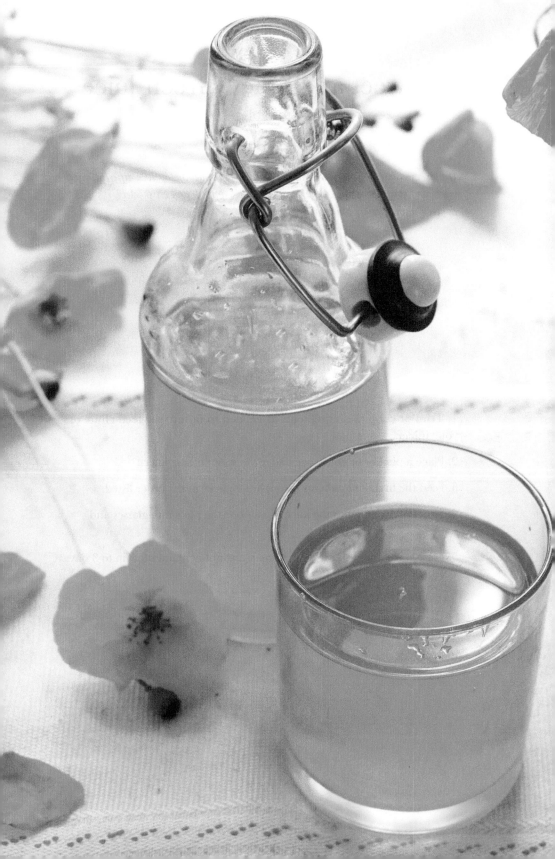

Sweet and Spicy Green Juice

MAKES 2 TO 3 SERVINGS, 8 TO 10 OUNCES EACH

If you are a fan of green juices but are looking for something a little different, try this sweet and spicy green juice. Made with luscious spinach and crisp celery, it's also flavored with celeriac, pear, and garlic.

1 BUNCH OR 2 CUPS SPINACH LEAVES
2 LARGE STALKS CELERY
1 MEDIUM APPLE
1 MEDIUM PEAR
1 SMALL BULB CELERIAC
1 GARLIC CLOVE, PEELED
PINCH OF CAYENNE PEPPER

1. Trim or chop the ingredients as needed to fit into the feed chute of your juicer.

2. Place a pitcher or container under the spout of the juicer.

3. Feed the first 6 ingredients through the juicer in the order listed.

4. Stir the cayenne into the juice; then pour the juice into glasses and serve immediately.

5. Fresh juice may be refrigerated in an airtight container for up to 3 days.

Go-Go Grapefruit Juice

Grapefruit juice on its own can sometimes be bitter, but when combined with fresh vegetables and ginger, it's absolutely delicious.

3 MEDIUM GRAPEFRUITS, HALVED AND PEELED
1 LARGE LEAF KALE
1 MEDIUM ENGLISH CUCUMBER
½ INCH GINGERROOT
PINCH OF GROUND CARDAMOM

1. Trim or chop the ingredients as needed to fit into the feed chute of your juicer.

2. Place a pitcher or container under the spout of the juicer.

3. Feed the first 4 ingredients through the juicer in the order listed.

4. Stir the cardamom into the juice; then pour the juice into glasses and serve immediately.

5. Fresh juice may be refrigerated in an airtight container for up to 3 days.

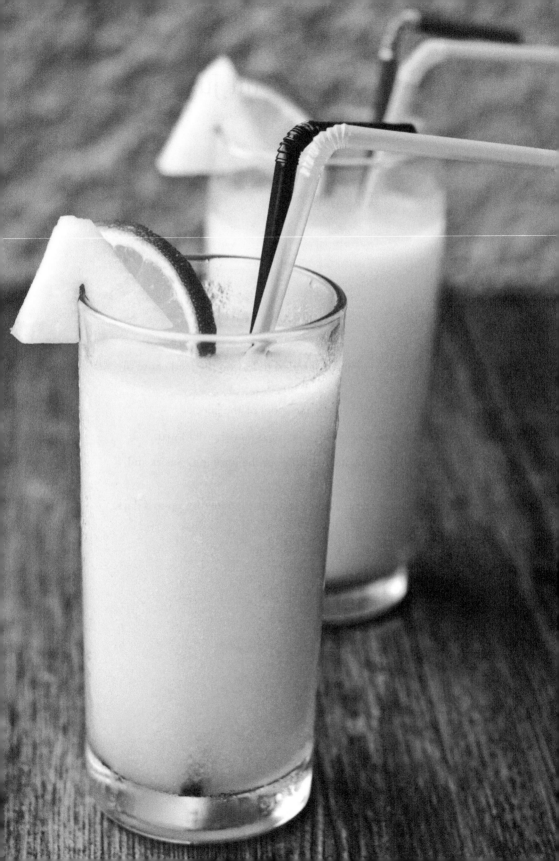

Lean Mean Green Juice Blend

Though low in calories, this juice blend packs quite a powerful punch. The green chili and jalapeño peppers give it a kick your taste buds won't be expecting.

1 BUNCH OR 2 CUPS ROMAINE LETTUCE
1 CUP STRAWBERRIES
1 SMALL GREEN CHILI PEPPER
½ SMALL JALAPEÑO, SEEDED
3 TO 4 SPRIGS FRESH CILANTRO

1. Trim or chop the ingredients as needed to fit into the feed chute of your juicer.

2. Place a pitcher or container under the spout of the juicer.

3. Feed the ingredients through the juicer in the order listed.

4. Stir the juice briefly; then pour it into glasses and serve immediately.

5. Fresh juice may be refrigerated in an airtight container for up to 3 days.

Hot Spiced Nectarine Juice

MAKES 3 SERVINGS, 8 TO 10 OUNCES EACH

A unique twist on apple cider, this juice is made with ripe nectarines and cantaloupe, flavored with a hint of lemon, nutmeg, and fresh ginger. In case that's not enough, it also has a pinch of cayenne pepper.

3 NECTARINES
1 SMALL CANTALOUPE, RIND REMOVED
1 LEMON, HALVED AND PEELED
1 INCH GINGERROOT
PINCH OF GROUND NUTMEG
PINCH OF CAYENNE PEPPER

1. Trim or chop the ingredients as needed to fit into the feed chute of your juicer.

2. Place a pitcher or container under the spout of the juicer.

3. Feed the first 4 ingredients through the juicer in the order listed.

4. Stir the nutmeg and cayenne into the juice; then pour the juice into a small saucepan.

5. Heat the juice until just steaming and serve immediately.

6. Fresh juice may be refrigerated in an airtight container for up to 3 days; do not save juice that has been heated.

Indian-Style Green Mango Juice

MAKES 2 SERVINGS, 8 TO 10 OUNCES EACH

If you're looking for something a little out of the ordinary, try this Indian-style green mango juice. Flavored with turmeric and ground cumin, it's like nothing you've tried before.

1 LARGE GREEN MANGO, PITTED

2½ CUPS COLD WATER

1 TEASPOON GROUND CUMIN

¼ TEASPOON FRESHLY GROUND PEPPER

PINCH OF TURMERIC

MINT LEAVES, FOR GARNISH

1. Trim or chop the mango as needed to fit into the feed chute of your juicer.

2. Place a pitcher or container under the spout of the juicer.

3. Feed the mango through the juicer.

4. Stir the water, cumin, pepper, and turmeric into the mango juice; then pour the juice into glasses.

5. Garnish with fresh mint leaves to serve.

6. Fresh juice may be refrigerated in an airtight container for up to 3 days.

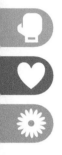

Spicy Carrot Ginger Juice

MAKES 2 SERVINGS, 8 TO 10 OUNCES EACH

Carrots are full of essential vitamins and minerals, including vitamin C to give your immune system a boost. If you aren't a fan of plain carrot juice, this recipe incorporates the flavors of grapefruit and ginger to make it unique.

6 LARGE CARROTS
2 MEDIUM GRAPEFRUITS, HALVED AND PEELED
1 LARGE STALK CELERY
1 INCH GINGERROOT
1 GARLIC CLOVE, PEELED
PINCH OF CAYENNE PEPPER

1. Trim or chop the ingredients as needed to fit into the feed chute of your juicer.

2. Place a pitcher or container under the spout of the juicer.

3. Feed the first 5 ingredients through the juicer in the order listed.

4. Stir the cayenne pepper into the juice; then pour it into glasses and serve immediately.

5. Fresh juice may be refrigerated in an airtight container for up to 3 days.

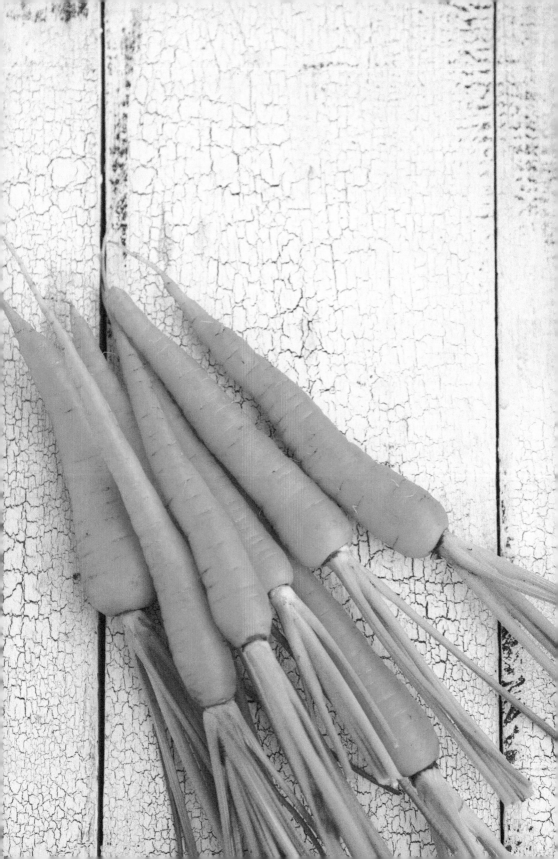

Red-Hot V-6 Juice

This spicy vegetable juice is loaded with flavor, not to mention essential vitamins and minerals. It gets its name from the six nutrient-packed ingredients.

2 LARGE STALKS CELERY
1 LARGE TOMATO
1 JALAPEÑO, SEEDED
½ LEMON, PEELED
¼ MEDIUM ENGLISH CUCUMBER
PINCH OF CAYENNE PEPPER

1. Trim or chop the ingredients as needed to fit into the feed chute of your juicer.

2. Place a pitcher or container under the spout of the juicer.

3. Feed the first 5 ingredients through the juicer in the order listed.

4. Stir the cayenne pepper into the juice; then pour the juice into glasses and serve immediately.

5. Fresh juice may be refrigerated in an airtight container for up to 3 days.

Raw Spiced Lemonade

This spiced lemonade is the ultimate cleansing detox drink. Gulp it down to feel refreshed after a long day, or after a tough workout to cool yourself down.

4 LEMONS, HALVED AND PEELED
2 CUPS COLD WATER
2 TABLESPOONS RAW HONEY (OPTIONAL)
½ TEASPOON BLACK SALT

1. Chop the lemons as needed to fit into the feed chute of your juicer.

2. Place a pitcher or container under the spout of the juicer.

3. Feed the lemons through the juicer.

4. Stir the water, honey (if using), and black salt into the lemon juice; then pour the juice into glasses and serve immediately.

5. Fresh juice may be refrigerated in an airtight container for up to 3 days.

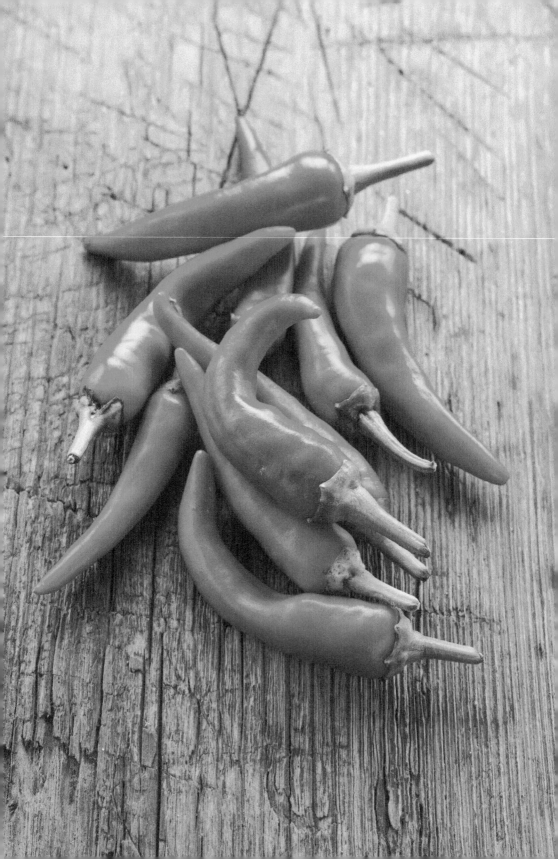

Cayenne Red Pepper Juice Blend

MAKES 2 TO 3 SERVINGS, 8 TO 10 OUNCES EACH

For this recipe you can choose whatever type of chili pepper you like. If you don't want the juice to get too spicy, use a green poblano pepper. If you're feeling adventurous, try a red serrano pepper or even a Thai chili.

2 MEDIUM RED BELL PEPPERS
2 SMALL CHILI PEPPERS
1 SMALL HEAD ROMAINE LETTUCE
1 SMALL STALK CELERY
PINCH OF CAYENNE PEPPER

1. Trim or cut the ingredients as needed to fit into the feed chute of your juicer.

2. Place a pitcher or container under the spout of the juicer.

3. Feed the first 4 ingredients through the juicer in the order listed.

4. Stir the cayenne pepper into the juice; then pour the juice into glasses and serve immediately.

5. Fresh juice may be refrigerated in an airtight container for up to 3 days.

Spicy Sunrise Juice Blend

This spicy blend is just the thing you need to wake you up in the morning. Full of fresh fruit flavor with a hint of heat, you'll be ready and raring to go in no time.

2 BLOOD ORANGES, HALVED AND PEELED
2 LARGE STALKS CELERY
1 LARGE NAVEL ORANGE, HALVED AND PEELED
1 MEDIUM GRAPEFRUIT, HALVED AND PEELED
1 KIWI, PEELED
½ INCH GINGERROOT
PINCH OF CAYENNE PEPPER

1. Trim or chop the ingredients as needed to fit into the feed chute of your juicer.

2. Place a pitcher or container under the spout of the juicer.

3. Feed the first 6 ingredients through the juicer in the order listed.

4. Stir the cayenne into the juice; then pour the juice into glasses and serve immediately.

5. Fresh juice may be refrigerated in an airtight container for up to 3 days.

Tart and Tangy Tomato Juice

Unless you're well versed in your citrus fruits, you may never have even heard of kumquats. These little orange fruits are packed with vitamins A, C, and E, not to mention omega-3 and omega-6 fatty acids.

2 LARGE TOMATOES
1 PINT KUMQUATS
½ LEMON, PEELED

1. Trim or chop the ingredients as needed to fit into the feed chute of your juicer.

2. Place a pitcher or container under the spout of the juicer.

3. Feed the ingredients through the juicer in the order listed.

4. Stir the juice briefly; then pour it into glasses and serve immediately.

5. Fresh juice may be refrigerated in an airtight container for up to 3 days.

Spiced Apple Pie Juice

There are many different types of apple, but one of the preferred varieties for pie is the Granny Smith. Granny Smith apples are crisp but not too sweet, as you will taste for yourself in this recipe!

4 MEDIUM GRANNY SMITH APPLES
1 TEASPOON APPLE CIDER VINEGAR
¾ TEASPOON GROUND CINNAMON
PINCH OF GROUND NUTMEG
1 SMALL SWEET APPLE, THINLY SLICED, FOR GARNISH
2 SMALL CINNAMON STICKS, FOR GARNISH

1. Trim or cut the Granny Smith apples as needed to fit into the feed chute of your juicer.

2. Place a pitcher or container under the spout of the juicer.

3. Feed the Granny Smith apples through the juicer.

4. Stir the apple cider vinegar, ground cinnamon, and nutmeg into the juice.

5. Pour the juice into 2 glasses, and garnish with the thinly sliced apple and a cinnamon stick to serve.

6. Fresh juice may be refrigerated in an airtight container for up to 3 days.

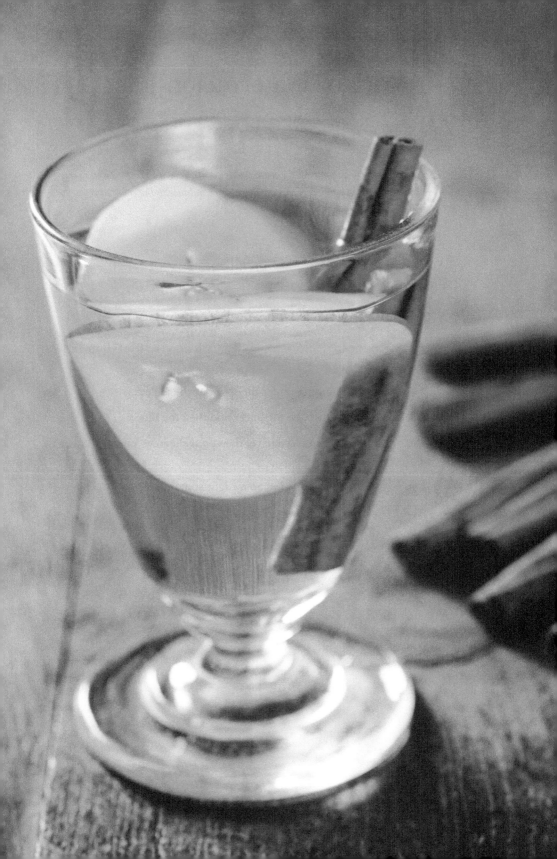

Wasabi Watermelon Juice

Wasabi is known for being one of the hottest condiments, and it is traditionally served with sushi. In this recipe, however, it provides a spicy balance to the cool, sweet flavor of watermelon.

1 LARGE SEEDLESS WATERMELON, RIND REMOVED
1 SMALL LIME, HALVED AND PEELED
½ TEASPOON WASABI POWDER

1. Trim or chop the ingredients as needed to fit into the feed chute of your juicer.

2. Place a pitcher or container under the spout of the juicer.

3. Feed the watermelon through the juicer and then the lime.

4. Stir the wasabi powder into the juice; then pour the juice into glasses and serve immediately.

5. Fresh juice may be refrigerated in an airtight container for up to 3 days.

Spicy Apple Detox Tonic

MAKES 2 TO 3 SERVINGS, 8 TO 10 OUNCES EACH

If you think you know apple juice, think again. This spicy apple tonic is like no apple juice you've ever tried. Drink it once and you'll never go back.

4 LARGE APPLES

2 LARGE STALKS CELERY

½ BUNCH OR 1 CUP SPINACH LEAVES

½ INCH GINGERROOT

PINCH OF CAYENNE PEPPER

1. Trim or chop the ingredients as needed to fit into the feed chute of your juicer.

2. Place a pitcher or container under the spout of the juicer.

3. Feed the first 4 ingredients through the juicer in the order listed.

4. Stir the cayenne into the juice; then pour the juice into glasses and serve immediately.

5. Fresh juice may be refrigerated in an airtight container for up to 3 days.

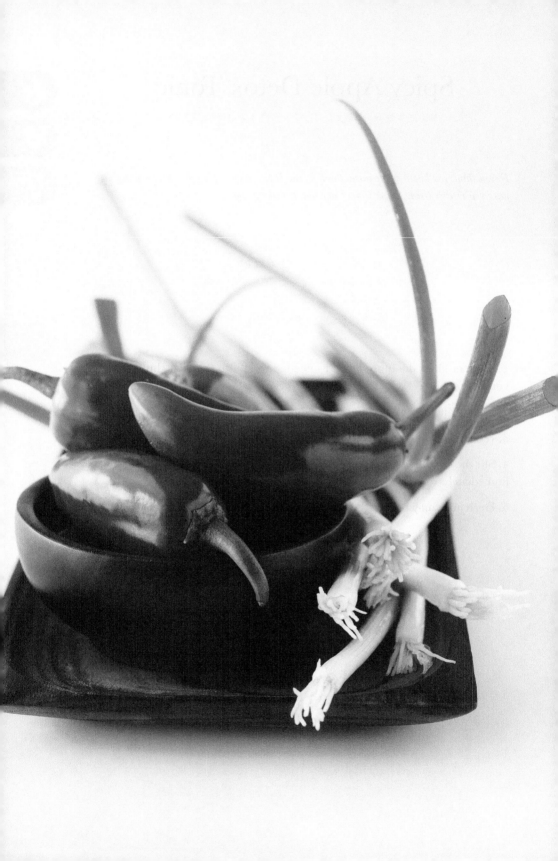

Jalapeño Hangover Juice Blend

After a night of drinking, your body is bound to be dehydrated. In this recipe you'll find ingredients that are full of water and essential nutrients to get you back to feeling your best.

2 MEDIUM PLUM TOMATOES
2 LARGE STALKS CELERY
2 MEDIUM SCALLIONS
1 MEDIUM JALAPEÑO, SEEDED
1 SMALL SEEDLESS CUCUMBER
½ INCH GINGERROOT

1. Trim or chop the ingredients as needed to fit into the feed chute of your juicer.

2. Place a pitcher or container under the spout of the juicer.

3. Feed the ingredients through the juicer in the order listed.

4. Stir the juice briefly; then pour it into glasses and serve immediately.

5. Fresh juice may be refrigerated in an airtight container for up to 3 days.

Pineapple Orange with a Kick

If you're tired of drinking the same old orange juice every morning, this pineapple-orange combo with a kick might be just the thing you've been looking for. Not only does it include the flavor of pineapple to shake things up, but the fresh flavor of cilantro and the kick of cayenne pepper are sure to get you going.

2 NAVEL ORANGES, PEELED AND HALVED
1 LARGE CARROT
½ PINEAPPLE, CORED AND HUSKED
½ LIME, PEELED
2 TO 3 SPRIGS FRESH CILANTRO
PINCH OF CAYENNE PEPPER

1. Trim or chop the ingredients as needed to fit into the feed chute of your juicer.

2. Place a pitcher or container under the spout of the juicer.

3. Feed the first 5 ingredients through the juicer in the order listed.

4. Stir the cayenne into the juice; then pour the juice into glasses and serve immediately.

5. Fresh juice may be refrigerated in an airtight container for up to 3 days.

Fiery Fig Mango Juice

Figs are not a part of many people's daily dietary routine. If you've never tried figs before, now's a great time to start. Figs have a sweet flavor and provide a number of significant health benefits, including reducing blood pressure and promoting healthy bone density.

8 SMALL FIGS, HALVED
2 MEDIUM MANGOS, PITTED
1 LARGE STALK CELERY
1 LARGE CARROT
1 JALAPEÑO, SEEDED
1 GARLIC CLOVE, PEELED
PINCH OF CAYENNE PEPPER

1. Trim or chop the ingredients as needed to fit into the feed chute of your juicer.

2. Place a pitcher or container under the spout of the juicer.

3. Feed the first 6 ingredients through the juicer in the order listed.

4. Stir the cayenne into the juice; then pour the juice into glasses and serve immediately.

5. Fresh juice may be refrigerated in an airtight container for up to 3 days.

Jump-Start Jicama Juice

MAKES 2 SERVINGS, 8 TO 10 OUNCES EACH

Jicama is technically a root and is also known by the name "yam bean." It's starchy and crisp, which makes for a cool and refreshing beverage.

3 LARGE CARROTS
2 CUPS CHOPPED JICAMA
1 MEDIUM BARTLETT PEAR
½ INCH GINGERROOT
PINCH OF CAYENNE PEPPER

1. Trim or chop the ingredients as needed to fit into the feed chute of your juicer.

2. Place a pitcher or container under the spout of the juicer.

3. Feed the first 4 ingredients through the juicer in the order listed.

4. Stir the cayenne pepper into the juice; then pour the juice into glasses and serve immediately.

5. Fresh juice may be refrigerated in an airtight container for up to 3 days.

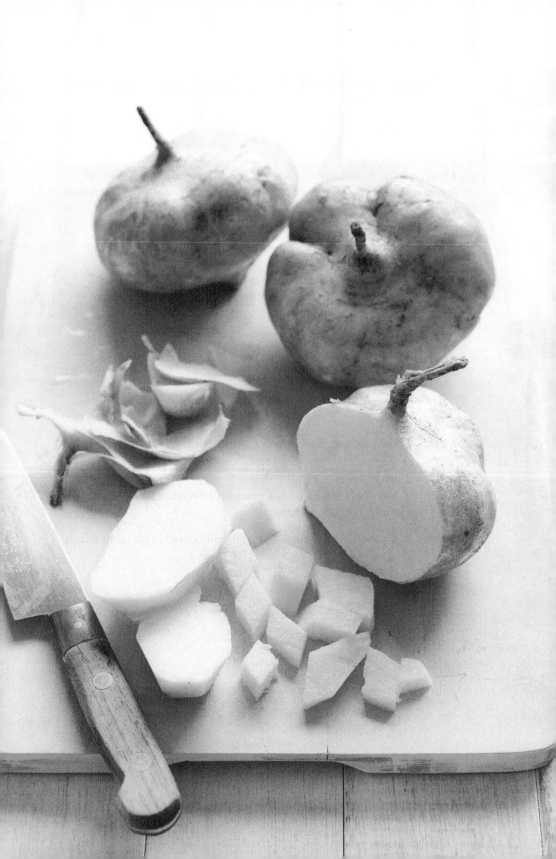

Raving Red Radish Juice Blend

Though radishes are rich with vitamins and minerals, the surprisingly healthful ingredient in this recipe is chlorella powder. Chlorella is a type of algae that contains high amounts of protein—as much as 5 grams per teaspoon!

6 MEDIUM RADISHES, GREENS INCLUDED
2 LARGE STALKS CELERY
2 SMALL PLUM TOMATOES
1 SMALL ZUCCHINI
1 TABLESPOON CHLORELLA POWDER
DASH OF HOT SAUCE

1. Trim or chop the ingredients as needed to fit into the feed chute of your juicer.

2. Place a pitcher or container under the spout of the juicer.

3. Feed the first 4 ingredients through the juicer in the order listed.

4. Stir the chlorella powder and hot sauce into the juice; then pour the juice into glasses and serve immediately.

5. Fresh juice may be refrigerated in an airtight container for up to 3 days.

Spicy Alkaline Juice Mixer

MAKES 3 SERVINGS, 8 TO 10 OUNCES EACH

In its healthiest state, your body should be slightly alkaline—a pH between 7.35 and 7.45 is optimal. The vegetables and herbs included in this recipe are known for their alkalinizing effects.

3 LARGE CARROTS

1 MEDIUM ENGLISH CUCUMBER

1 SMALL BULB FENNEL, STALK INCLUDED

½ BUNCH OR 1 CUP KALE

¼ CUP FRESH BASIL LEAVES, PACKED

1 INCH GINGERROOT

1. Trim or chop the ingredients as needed to fit into the feed chute of your juicer.

2. Place a pitcher or container under the spout of the juicer.

3. Feed the ingredients through the juicer in the order listed.

4. Stir the juice briefly; then pour it into glasses and serve immediately.

5. Fresh juice may be refrigerated in an airtight container for up to 3 days.

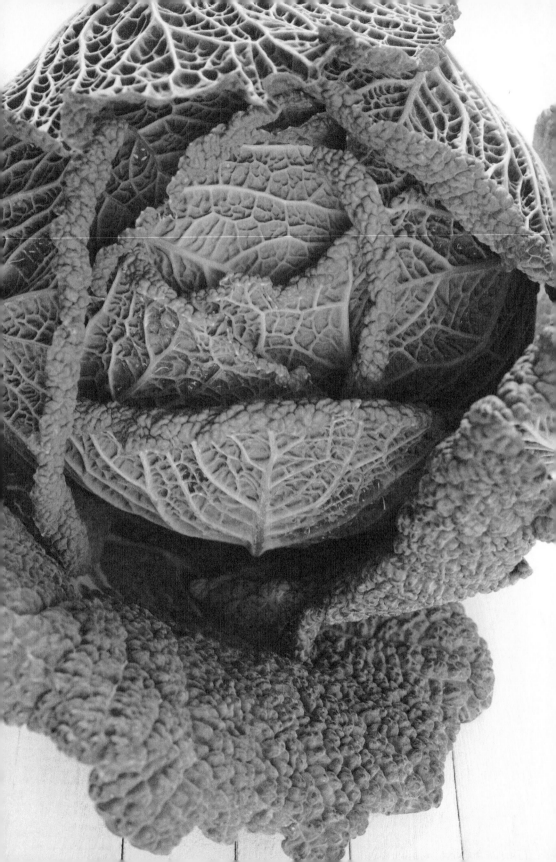

Savory Spring Green Juice

Also known as curly cabbage, savoy cabbage has ruffled, almost lacy leaves. This cabbage is very tender with a fresh flavor that works well in this recipe.

1 SMALL HEAD SAVOY CABBAGE
1 CUP BABY SPINACH LEAVES
1 CUP CHOPPED COLLARD GREENS
1 SMALL BEET, GREENS INCLUDED

1. Trim or cut the ingredients as needed to fit into the feed chute of your juicer.

2. Place a pitcher or container under the spout of the juicer.

3. Feed the ingredients through the juicer in the order listed.

4. Stir the juice briefly; then pour it into glasses and serve immediately.

5. Fresh juice may be refrigerated in an airtight container for up to 3 days.

Glossary

Antioxidants: Molecules that prevent other molecules from oxidizing. They protect cells from free radical damage and may also help prevent cancer and other chronic diseases.

Centrifugal juicer: A juicer that uses a grated basket that acts as a spinning blade, grinding the produce and extracting the juice.

Cold-pressed juice: Juice extracted with minimal heat production, which destroys enzymes; usually juice created with a masticating juicer.

Coumarins: A type of anti-cancer compound shown to help repair cellular damage caused by free radicals.

Detoxification: The process of removing harmful substances from the body.

Enzymes: Substances produced by the body that help catalyze biochemical processes.

Juice cleanse: A regimen in which an individual receives all of his or her daily nutrition from fruit and vegetable juices.

Juicing: The act of extracting liquid (juice) from plant tissues, mainly fresh fruits and vegetables. Juicing can also refer to a dietary habit of consuming nutrients and calories in the form of fresh-squeezed juice as an alternative or supplement to solid foods.

Macronutrients: Nutrients the human body needs in the largest quantities, including protein, carbohydrate, and fats.

Masticating juicer: A motor-driven juicer that operates more slowly than a centrifugal juicer. Masticating juicers work by kneading and grinding the material in the feed chute, squeezing the juice out into a container.

Micronutrients: Nutrients required by the human body in small quantities to maintain healthful physiological function, including vitamins, minerals, phytochemicals, and trace elements.

Probiotics: Live bacteria that serve to regulate and improve digestion.

Pulp: The fibrous plant matter left over after juicing.

Supplement: Something added to the diet to make up for a deficiency, such as a pill or capsule containing vitamins, minerals, or other nutrients.

Triturating juicer: Also called a twin-gear juicer, it utilizes a two-step juicing process; produce is fed through the juicer to be crushed and then pressed.

Toxin: A harmful substance that can cause serious health problems, even in small doses.

APPENDIX A

Fruit and Vegetable Nutrition Charts

FRUITS FOR JUICING SERVING SIZE = 100 GRAMS

FOOD	CALORIES	PROTEIN (G)	CARBS (G)	FATS (G)	FIBER (G)
Apple	50	0.26	13.8	0.17	2.4
Apricot	48	1.00	11.0	0.00	2.0
Blackberries	43	1.39	9.6	0.49	5.3
Blood orange	50	0.00	11.0	0.00	2.0
Blueberries	57	0.74	14.5	0.33	2.4
Cantaloupe	34	0.84	8.6	0.19	0.9
Cherries	50	1.00	12.2	0.30	1.6
Cranberries	46	0.00	12.0	0.00	5.0
Figs	74	1.00	19.0	0.00	3.0
Gooseberries	44	1.00	10.0	1.00	4.0
Grapes	69	0.72	18.0	0.16	0.9
Grapefruit	42	0.77	10.7	0.14	1.7
Guava	68	3.00	14.0	1.00	5.0
Honeydew	36	1.00	9.0	0.00	1.0
Jicama	38	1.00	9.0	0.00	5.0
Kiwi	61	1.00	14.6	0.52	3.0
Kumquat	71	2.00	16.0	1.00	6.0
Lemon	29	1.10	9.3	0.30	2.8
Lime	30	1.00	11.0	0.00	3.0

FOOD	CALORIES	PROTEIN (G)	CARBS (G)	FATS (G)	FIBER (G)
Mango	70	0.50	17.0	0.27	1.8
Nectarine	44	1.00	11.0	0.00	2.0
Orange	47	0.94	11.7	0.12	2.4
Papaya	39	0.61	9.8	0.14	1.8
Passion fruit	97	2.20	23.4	0.70	10.4
Peach	39	0.91	9.5	0.25	1.5
Pear	58	0.38	13.8	0.12	3.1
Persimmon	127	1.00	33.0	0.00	0.0
Pineapple	50	0.54	13.5	0.12	1.4
Plum	46	1.00	11.0	0.00	1.0
Pomegranate	83	1.67	18.7	1.17	4.0
Raspberries	52	1.20	11.9	0.65	6.5
Starfruit	31	1.00	7.0	0.00	3.0
Strawberries	32	0.67	7.7	0.30	2.0
Tangerine	53	0.81	13.3	0.31	1.8
Watermelon	30	1.00	8.0	0.00	0.0

VEGETABLES FOR JUICING SERVING SIZE = 100 GRAMS

FOOD	CALORIES	PROTEIN (G)	CARBS (G)	FATS (G)	FIBER (G)
Arugula	25	2.58	3.65	0.66	1.6
Asparagus	20	2.20	3.38	0.12	2.1
Beets	45	1.61	9.56	0.17	2.8
Bell pepper	31	0.99	6.03	0.30	2.1
Bok Choy	13	1.50	2.18	0.20	1.0
Broccoli	34	2.82	6.64	0.37	2.6
Brussels sprouts	43	3.38	8.95	0.30	3.8
Cabbage	25	1.30	5.80	0.10	2.5
Carrots	41	0.93	9.58	0.24	2.8
Cauliflower	25	1.92	4.97	0.28	2.0
Celeriac	42	1.00	9.00	0.00	2.0
Celery	16	1.00	3.00	0.00	2.0
Collard greens	30	2.45	5.69	0.42	3.6
Cucumber	15	0.65	3.63	0.11	0.5
Dandelion greens	45	3.00	9.00	1.00	4.0
Kale	50	3.30	10.00	0.70	2.0
Kohlrabi	27	2.00	6.00	0.00	4.0
Mustard greens	26	3.00	5.00	0.00	3.0
Onion	40	1.00	9.00	0.00	2.0
Parsnips	75	1.20	18.00	0.30	4.9
Pumpkin	26	1.00	6.50	0.10	0.5
Radishes	16	1.00	3.00	0.00	2.0
Romaine lettuce	15	1.36	2.79	0.15	1.3
Rutabaga	36	1.00	8.00	0.00	3.0

FOOD	CALORIES	PROTEIN (G)	CARBS (G)	FATS (G)	FIBER (G)
Scallions	32	2.00	7.00	0.00	3.0
Spinach	23	2.86	3.63	0.39	2.2
Sugar snap peas	42	3.00	8.00	0.00	3.0
Summer squash	16	1.00	3.00	0.00	1.0
Sweet potato	86	1.60	20.10	0.05	3.0
Swiss chard	19	3.27	3.74	0.20	1.6
Tomatoes	18	0.90	3.90	0.20	1.2
Turnip	32	1.00	7.00	0.00	3.0
Turnip greens	32	1.00	7.00	0.00	3.0
Wheatgrass	23	2.00	3.00	0.00	0.0
Zucchini	17	1.21	3.11	0.32	1.0

7-Day Quick Cleanse Guidelines

Juice fasts are becoming more popular as a way to "cleanse" the body and reset physiological processes that have been riddled with pollutants, toxins, and food laced with preservatives. Many people go on a juice fast hoping that it will be a quick fix to their weight and health problems. Instead, it's best to think of juicing as a "gateway drug" to better health and clean eating.

—JONATHAN BECHTEL, *LIVING GREEN MAGAZINE*

Incorporating fresh fruit and vegetable juices into your daily routine is a great way to get your health on track. If you're used to a diet loaded with processed foods, artificial ingredients, and refined sugars, your body may be in rough shape, even if you feel fine. You may not realize just how much better you can feel until you have cleansed your body of accumulated toxins and gotten yourself into some healthier habits. As with any big dietary change, you should consult a medical professional before beginning. In this section you'll find guidelines for a quick, seven-day cleanse to help you start your juicing journey off right.

Before You Start

As long as you already have a juicer, the only other things you need to worry about before starting your cleanse are the ingredients for your juice. The beauty of a juice cleanse is that you don't necessarily need to use recipes—you can simply stock up on fresh produce and then use a variety of fruits and vegetables to create your daily juices. Keep in mind that different fruits and vegetables contain different nutrients, so it's important that you switch things up, trying out different ingredients as you go along.

Quick Juice Cleanse Guidelines

If you perform a simple online search for "juice cleanse," you'll find a number of results for companies that specialize in creating customized juice cleanse plans. The benefit of these companies is that you can purchase the juices directly and follow a set plan for a predetermined number of days. The downside to this is that they can be expensive. Many juice cleanses cost between fifty and seventy-five dollars a day. For the same price you would pay for a single day's worth of commercial juice, you can buy several days' worth of fresh produce to make your own.

The most important thing you need to remember if you hope to succeed in your seven-day juice cleanse is that you should try to stick to a regular schedule to avoid hunger. You don't necessarily need to sip juice throughout the entire day, but you should plan to drink six to eight juices (12 to 18 ounces each) to keep your hunger at bay. Don't be conservative with the amount of juice you drink in the morning, as this can result in headaches or other negative side effects. Do whatever works for you. For many people, it works best to sip the juice slowly, letting each juice last about one hour and waiting twenty to thirty minutes before beginning the next serving of juice.

If you're not inclined to create your own juices from scratch, feel free to use the recipes in this book. All you need to do is pick out six or seven juice recipes for each day of your cleanse. To make things easier on yourself (and on your wallet) try to stick to simple recipes for midmorning and afternoon snacks. These recipes should include no more than three ingredients. For a seven-day cleanse, it's recommended that you pick three or four different recipes and rotate through them as needed. For your three main meals of the day (breakfast, lunch, and dinner), choose juices that incorporate a variety of ingredients. If you plan to use recipes from this book, be sure to draw equally from the Green Juices, Fruit Juices, and Vegetable Juices sections. You may even want to incorporate some of the recipes from the Savory and Spicy Juices section as well.

Keep in mind that no two people will react to a juice cleanse the same way. Some individuals may have no problem making it through an entire seven-day cleanse, while for others, three days in a row may be a struggle. As you engage in your cleanse, pay attention to your body and consider keeping a journal of your mood and physical reactions. If the cleanse makes you feel tired, irritable, or sluggish to the point where it's interfering with your work or life, you may want to cut the cleanse short. Another option is to swap out one juice meal per day for a real meal. If you choose this option, your best bet is to make dinner a real meal, basing it on fresh vegetables and lean protein.

Daily Tips to Follow

While engaging in your seven-day cleanse, these tips may help get you through the challenging times. You needn't be concerned if you experienced headaches for the first day or two. Don't worry—the side effects should go away and soon you will be feeling just like new.

- Try drinking a glass of lemon water first thing in the morning.

- Drink at least 16 ounces of water after each juice meal to stay hydrated.

- Each juice should consist of between 12 and 18 ounces.

- Drink your juices slowly to optimize the absorption of nutrients.

- Drink your last juice about two to three hours before bedtime.

- Engage in moderate daily exercise, like walking, during your cleanse.

- Try to incorporate some stress-relieving exercises during your cleanse to detoxify your mind as well as your body.

Note: Though you may see juice cleanses recommended as a way to lose weight quickly, you should not rely on them for this result. You may lose weight during a juice cleanse, but it's likely to be water weight that may return quickly if you go back to poor eating habits after the cleanse. To get the most out of your juice cleanse, think of it as a transition into a healthier routine, a means of detoxifying your body to create a clean slate for your journey into juicing.

References

Bechtel, Jonathan. "Juice Fasting for Beginners: The Cleanse that Energizes." *Living Green Magazine*. January 2, 2013. http://livinggreenmag.com /2013/01/02/food-health/juice-fasting-for-beginners-the-cleanse -that-energizes/.

Bridgeford, Callum. "Juicing for Health." *Energise for Life*. Accessed September 15, 2013. http://www.energiseforlife.com/juicing.php.

Brooks, Sarah. "Healthy Benefits of Spicy Foods." *SheKnows*. March 21, 2013. http://www.sheknows.com/food-and-recipes/articles/988185 /health-benefits-of-spicy-foods.

Calbom, Cherie. *The Juice Lady's Big Book of Juices and Green Smoothies*. Lake Mary, FL: Siloam, 2013.

Cross, Joe. "Fat, Sick and Nearly Dead: How One Man Took Control of His Eating Habits." *Huffington Post*. November 29, 2010. http://www.huffingtonpost.com/joe-cross/fat-sick-and-nearly-dead -_b_789298.html.

Cross, Joe. "Why Juice." *Reboot with Joe*. Accessed September 15, 2013. http://www.rebootwithjoe.com/juicing/benefits/.

Dietetics Department. *Vitamins and Minerals Chart*. Singapore: National University Hospital, 2006. http://www.nuh.com.sg/wbn/slot/u1753 /Patients%20and%20Visitors/Specialities/Pharmacy/Health%20 Supplements/HSL_VitaminMineral.pdf.

Drake, Victoria J. "Nutrition and Immunity, Part I." Linus Pauling Institute Research Newsletter, Spring/Summer 2010. http://lpi.oregonstate.edu /ss10/nutrition.html.

FDA.gov. "Nutrition Information for Raw Fruits, Vegetables and Fish." Accessed September 15, 2013. http://www.fda.gov/food /ingredientspackaginglabeling/labelingnutrition/ucm063367.htm.

Fern's Nutrition. "Juicers: 5 Main Types of Juicers." Accessed September 15, 2013. http://www.fernsnutrition.com/juicer_types.htm.

FitDay. "The Nutrition of Fruit Juice." Accessed September 15, 2013. http://www.fitday.com/fitness-articles/nutrition/healthy-eating /the-nutrition-of-fruit-juice.html.

Food Matters. "2013 Juicer Buying Guide." Accessed September 15, 2013. http://foodmatters.tv/juicer-buying-guide.

Foster, Cynthia. "The Healing Power of Juicing." EatVeg.com. Accessed September 15, 2013. http://www.eatveg.com/powerofjuicing.html.

Fuhrman, Joel. *Super Immunity: The Essential Nutrition Guide for Boosting Your Body's Defenses to Live Longer, Stronger, and Disease Free.* New York: HarperOne, 2011.

Guadagno, Maria. "The Benefits of Detoxing." Bombshellblueprint.com. Accessed September 17, 2013. http://bombshellblueprint.com /2013/04/the-benefits-of-detoxing/

Harvest Essentials, "Which Juicer Is Right for You?" Accessed September 15, 2013. http://www.harvestessentials.com/whatjuicisri.html.

Healthy Juicer. "Health Benefits of Juicing." Accessed September 15, 2013. http://www.healthyjuicer.com/health-benefits-of-juicing.html.

Hoffman, Ronald. "Nutrients That Boost Immunity." DrHoffman.com. Accessed September 15, 2013. http://www.drhoffman.com /page.cfm/125.

Juice Lane. "Cold Press." Accessed September 15, 2013. http://juicelane.com /cold_press.html.

Juice Master. "A–Z of Fruit and Vegetables." Accessed September 15, 2013. http://www.juicemaster.com/us/juice-therapy/a-to-z.

Ko, Lisa. "5 Things You Need to Know about . . . Juicing." *Need to Know.* August 11, 2011. http://www.pbs.org/wnet/need-to-know/health /juicing/10814/.

Living Greens. "Benefits." Accessed September 15, 2013. http://www.livinggreensjuice.com/Benefits-of-Juicing-s/1824.htm.

"Losing Weight." Centers for Disease Control and Prevention. Last modified August 17, 2011. http://www.cdc.gov/healthyweight/losing_weight/.

Ms. S. "Healthy Juice: There's Only One Type That's Worth Drinking!" The S File: Health. December 28, 2010. http://www.health.thesfile.com /healthy-juice-theres-only-one-type-thats-worth-drinking/.

Nelson, Jennifer K. "Is Juicing Healthier than Eating Whole Fruits and Vegetables?" Mayo Clinic. October 21, 2010. http://www.mayoclinic.com /health/juicing/AN02107.

Nguyen, Anna. "Juicing: How Healthy Is It?" WebMD. Last modified January 11, 2012. http://www.webmd.com/diet/features/juicing -health-risks-and-benefits.

Raw-Wisdom.com, "Juice Feasting Supplements and (Super)foods." Accessed September 15, 2013. http://www.raw-wisdom.com /jfsupplements.

Reboot with Joe. "A-Z Produce Prep: Fruits and Vegetables." Accessed September 15, 2013. http://www.rebootwithjoe.com/juicing /produce-prep/.

Simkins, Vanessa. "Guide for Using Herbs in Juice: Enhance Your Fresh Juice with Herbal Remedies." All About Juicing. Accessed September 15, 2013. http://www.all-about-juicing.com/Using-Herbs.html.

Simkins, Vanessa. "Juicing for Skin Conditions." All About Juicing. Accessed September 15, 2013. http://www.all-about-juicing.com /skin-conditions.html.

The Dr. Oz Show. "The Healing Properties of Juicing." May 1, 2013. http://www.doctoroz.com/videos/healing-properties-juicing.

The World's Healthiest Foods. Accessed September 15, 2013. Whfoods.org.

Tune, Michele L. "Raw Juice vs. Bottled." *RawPeople.com*. Accessed September 15, 2013. http://www.rawpeople.com/index.php?option =com_content&id=328&Itemid=110.

Wagner, Linda. "Juicing for Weight Loss." *Linda Wagner* (blog). June 14, 2012. http://lindawagner.net/blog/2012/06/juicing-for-weight-loss /index.html.

Young, Lisa. "Benefits of Fruits and Vegetables." *Huffington Post*. July 12, 2012. http://www.huffingtonpost.com/dr-lisa-young/healthy-food_b _1665279.html.

Index

CPSIA information can be obtained at www.ICGtesting.com
Printed in the USA
BVOW10s1829281013

334659BV00002B/2/P